T0177623

Everybody's War

EVERYBODY'S WAR

The Politics of Aid in the Syria Crisis

Edited by Jehan Bseiso, Michiel Hofman,
and Jonathan Whittall

With a foreword by Amani Ballour

OXFORD
UNIVERSITY PRESS

OXFORD
UNIVERSITY PRESS

Oxford University Press is a department of the University of Oxford. It furthers
the University's objective of excellence in research, scholarship, and education
by publishing worldwide. Oxford is a registered trade mark of Oxford University
Press in the UK and certain other countries.

Published in the United States of America by Oxford University Press
198 Madison Avenue, New York, NY 10016, United States of America.

© Médecins Sans Frontières 2021

Library of Congress Cataloging-in-Publication Data
Names: Bseiso, Jehan, editor. | Hofman, Michiel, editor. |
Whittall, Jonathan, editor. | Médecins Sans frontières (Association)
Title: Everybody's war : The Politics of Aid in the Syria Crisis / edited by Jehan Bseiso,
Michiel Hofman, and Jonathan Whittall.
Description: New York, NY : Oxford University Press, [2021] |
Includes bibliographical references and index. |
Identifiers: LCCN 2021008294 (print) | LCCN 2021008295 (ebook) |
ISBN 9780197514641 (hardback) | ISBN 9780197514665 (epub) |
ISBN 9780197514672 (online)
Subjects: MESH: Médecins sans frontières (Association) |
Relief Work | Armed Conflicts | Politics | Delivery of Health Care |
Voluntary Health Agencies | Syria
Classification: LCC HV555.S95 (print) | LCC HV555.S95 (ebook) |
NLM HV 555.S95 | DDC 338.91095691—dc23
LC record available at https://lccn.loc.gov/2021008294
LC ebook record available at https://lccn.loc.gov/2021008295

DOI: 10.1093/oso/9780197514641.001.0001

9 8 7 6 5 4 3 2

Printed by Sheridan Books, Inc., United States of America

CONTENTS

FOREWORD

From 2012 until 2018, I have been a doctor on the front lines of the war in Syria, working under siege and nonstop bombardment. When I was asked to write the foreword to this book on the politics of aid in Syria, I thought the best way to convey the topic's importance would be to describe my direct experiences: the patients I treated, the ones I couldn't save, and the inability or unwillingness of anybody to help us.

Maybe this is "everybody's war" in Syria, as this book's title suggests, but I am sure not everybody will pay the price.

SIEGE AND STARVATION IN EAST GHOUTA

Only thirty kilometers from Damascus, in the suburb of Eastern Ghouta an endless siege gripped the region, and children were left starving and sick as their parents desperately struggled to provide such basics of life as food, shelter, and medicine.

Working as a pediatrician in a besieged war zone was torture. Each day many children walked into my clinic with their mothers, and they often walked out with shattered hopes because of the lack of medication, diagnostic tools, and treatment.

Food and medication were prevented from entering Eastern Ghouta at the time, as peaceful protests erupted in the region, with demonstrators demanding essential rights and calling for a life of dignity. Similar uprisings occurred in many Syrian regions and cities. Alas, the Syrian people were to pay an incalculable price.

In response to the protests, the government destroyed hospitals, schools, markets, even kindergartens. Fathers, mothers, and children were killed, and to this day, many have not been found dead or alive. All kinds of weaponry were used against civilians; protesters were arrested, killed, and tortured.

Cancer patients and those who suffered from chronic illnesses died in front of me; we didn't even have painkillers to alleviate their suffering. No matter how much parents and doctors begged at checkpoints to allow the emergency medical evacuation of critical patients, very few trickled out, and most died of preventable and treatable conditions.

I was the head of the central hospital in the region. Getting our hands on basic medication and medical supplies—even for mild, treatable conditions—was incredibly challenging. We were forced to dig tunnels in order to smuggle medical equipment and medication. In areas controlled by the Syrian government, we purchased supplies from the merchants of war who exploited our desperation. Even then we couldn't get everything we needed.

My patients suffered from excruciating pain, illness, and wounds. Millions of children and adults also suffered from post-traumatic stress disorder and mental illnesses that will most likely accompany them for life.

Our hospital was built underground to protect it from the continuous, systematic shelling by the Syrian government and its foreign allies. We believed they targeted hospitals to thwart our efforts. We simply had opposing objectives: we wanted to live.

My hospital was bombed many times. One of the departments was completely destroyed, and three of our nurses were killed.

Pledging to ensure our safety, the United Nations asked us to share the GPS coordinates of our hospitals. After some of our colleagues succumbed to this request, Russian airplanes nevertheless bombarded their hospitals, blatantly disregarding international law, ethical values, and the rules of war. For us in East Ghouta, this was further proof of the United Nations' failure and inability to protect people.

"ASSAD, OR THE COUNTRY BURNS"

Syria is still burning. For over five years, in Eastern Ghouta, we witnessed thousands of brutal massacres against civilians and children.

I believe that in 2013, the Syrian government used internationally prohibited chemical weapons and murdered more than fifteen hundred people in one night, most of whom were hungry women and children.

That terrifying night, thousands of innocent people inhaled toxic gas and suffocated before our eyes. We couldn't help them.

I remember it as if it were yesterday. I woke in the middle of that night to find hundreds of bodies lying on the ground, suffocating, but wound-free.

A hundred others, most of whom were children, were fighting for their lives. Their lips were blue and their bodies were pale.

We did not have enough medication and medical equipment, and we had only a few doctors on our team along with some volunteers. We tried to save as many people as possible, but death was always faster than us.

One mother, a close acquaintance of mine, called me that night to tell me her three children had suffocated and died. One father implored me to save his only child. He had waited many years to be blessed with a son. The child instantly suffocated to death.

We saw many hungry children lose their families and homes due to the endless bombardments.

We treated thousands of injured patients, many of them with critical injuries. We saw children with amputated arms and legs. They repeatedly asked us to explain why this had happened to them, but we had no answers.

Once, a five-year-old child asked me why he had lost his hand. I remained silent.

" 'HELL ON EARTH' IN SYRIA'S EASTERN GHOUTA MUST END": THE UNITED NATIONS, FEBRUARY 26, 2018

Over the years, there was no shortage of statements and condemnations from the international community. But not one ever came close to describing the level of pain and horror suffered by a single child.

After thousands of innocent souls had been massacred using all kinds of weapons, the UN Security Council finally convened. We impatiently waited for measures that would save hungry and wounded children and patients. I told patients and their parents that the Security Council was to convene soon and find a solution. This was our only hope. But the Russian veto, shattered our dreams again and again, meeting after meeting. We were caught in the deadly grip of criminal action on the ground and criminal inaction in the corridors of power.

After the chemical massacre of 2013, one of the worst in modern history, the so-called international community confiscated the weapon, but they left the criminal on the loose.

The international community has let us down hundreds of times. They knew the truth and watched bodies torn and shredded on screen. They heard the bombs and warplanes; they heard the cries of the doctors who desperately asked for medication and medical equipment to rescue the wounded and treat patients. Their response to the besiegement of around half a million citizens was to send, every year or two, a convoy of medical and food supplies that would barely meet the needs of one neighborhood in East Ghouta. They submitted to the pressures exerted by the Syrian government; surgical kits, medical equipment, and anesthesia were not allowed to enter, children's milk was a prohibited item, and too often, humanitarian aid supplies were blocked or redirected, never to reach their destination.

The international community was only trying to deal with the consequences of the problem and respond to the humanitarian crisis, rather than solving the root issue.

In a particularly dark moment, I was forced to deprive hundreds of children of nutritional biscuits supplied by the United Nations in small quantities specifically meant for the malnourished only. The truth was that all the children in Ghouta were hungry, if not medically malnourished, and their parents took them to the hospital hoping they would get anything, even a slice of butter.

Our medical team examined and assessed each child, to preserve the limited quantity of food for those who were most in need. Consequently, hungry children who were not yet suffering from malnutrition did not receive any food and left the hospital with empty bellies.

My heart ached at the sight of parents gathered at the clinic door, hoping that their children would be diagnosed with malnutrition, only to leave later, disappointed to learn that their healthy child would sleep on an empty stomach for yet another day.

DEAD, DISAPPEARED, DROWNED, OR DISPLACED

For a decade, the world has borne silent witness to the agony of the Syrian people. Syrians continue to die unjustly today, from shelling or bombs, or through the denial of basic rights to medical care and food. Thousands are detained and disappeared in prisons where they have been brutally tortured for years, as depicted in the 2014 Syrian detainee report whose photographs shook the entire world but could not change anything on the ground.

More than half the Syrian population is homeless outside of Syria.

Hundreds of innocent Syrians drowned while trying to seek asylum, security, and dignity, and their bodies are still at sea. Why would a parent risk taking the "death boats" if not for the horror, killings, humiliation, and sheer misery of life in Syria?

Today, millions of Syrians are displaced, living in camps north of Syria and in neighboring countries, such as Lebanon and Jordan. The situation in these camps is very difficult; access to health care and food, education, and employment depends on intermittent aid and the growing weariness of states and host communities.

We continue to plead with the international community to protect Syrian civilians: men, women, and children who are not part of the war. But the medicine we need to truly heal is justice. That is my prescription. I only hope that my cries will not continue to go unheard.

Dr. Amani Ballour

ABOUT THE EDITORS

Jehan Bseiso is currently the Executive Director for Médecins Sans Frontières (MSF) Lebanon. She joined MSF in 2008 and worked in countries such as Afghanistan, Pakistan, Iraq, Ethiopia, Belgium, and elsewhere mostly in communications and advocacy. Also a researcher and a poet, she coedited the anthology *Making Mirrors: Writing/Righting by and from Refugees* published in 2019, as well as coauthored *I Remember My Name*, a Palestine Book Award-winning collection (2016). Jehan holds a Master of Arts in English Literature from the American University of Beirut.

Michiel Hofman worked for Médecins Sans Frontières (MSF) in field missions between 1993 and 1998 as Emergency Coordinator and Head of Mission for MSF in Liberia, Democratic Republic of Congo, Bosnia, Burundi, Sri Lanka, Brazil, South Sudan, and Kosovo, returning to his former career as freelance journalist in between missions. Between 1999 and 2001, Michiel cofounded The Antares Foundation, a Dutch nonprofit organization that supports local nongovernmental organizations (NGOs) in providing psychosocial support for staff working in high-stress environments. Michiel returned to MSF in 2001 working as Country Director in Russia, Director of Operations at MSF Amsterdam HQ, and as Country Representative for Afghanistan. Since 2011 Michiel works as senior humanitarian specialist for MSF based out of Belfast, concentrating on research, training, and operational support as well as publications in the humanitarian field. He was the coeditor of "The Politics of Fear," a book examining the Ebola response in West Africa (Oxford University Press, 2017).

Jonathan Whittall is Director of the Analysis department for Médecins Sans Frontières Operational Centre in Brussels. The Analysis Department conducts research, develops advocacy strategies, and provides strategic operational support on the thematics of migration and refugees, the politics of health, humanitarianism and conflict, and negotiated access. In this role, and in his prior role as Head of Humanitarian Analysis, Jonathan provided strategic support to MSF operations in conflict environments, including in Pakistan, Afghanistan, Iraq, South Sudan, and Syria. He previously established and headed the organization's Programmes Unit in his home town of Johannesburg. Following this he was an Emergency Coordinator in MSF's medical humanitarian responses in Libya, Bahrain, and Syria. He has contributed to academic journals and newspapers on the politics of humanitarian aid. He holds a Masters degree in Humanitarian Studies and a PhD from the Liverpool School of Tropical Medicine.

CONTRIBUTORS

Aula Abbara, MBBS, DTMH, MD(Res) is a consultant in Infectious Diseases/General Internal Medicine at Imperial College NHS Healthcare Trust, London and an Honorary Clinical Lecturer at Imperial College. She has volunteered in various humanitarian and refugee settings including Greece, Sierra Leone, Turkey, and Jordan, undertaking direct clinical work, teaching healthcare workers, and building capacity. Since 2012, she has volunteered predominantly with Syrian nongovernmental organizations. Her research interests include attacks on health care, antimicrobial resistance in conflict, refugee healthcare workers, and other interests more broadly relating to global and humanitarian health. Dr. Aula co-chairs the Syria Public Health Network, is the research lead for the Syrian American Medical Society, and is part of SyRG-LSHTM (Syrian Research Group at LSHTM.)

Amani Ballour was born and raised in the province of East Ghouta in Syria. She completed her general medical studies at the University of Damascus in 2012. She chose to abandon her medical specialization in Pediatrics in order to provide urgent medical care in East Ghouta at the onset of the war in Syria. For years, Dr. Amani has treated hundreds of children, many of them injured and wounded from bombing. In partnership with the King Baudouin Foundation, Dr. Amani recently established Al Amal Fund, which aims to support female leaders in conflict zones who face many critical challenges, and often defy deeply entrenched gender biases.

Dawn Chatty is Professor Emeritus of Anthropology and former Director of the Refugee Studies Centre (2011–2014) at Oxford University, where she still lectures. She is particularly interested in nomadic pastoral tribes, as well as the young people among refugees. She studied at the University of California in Los Angeles (UCLA) and Institute of Social Studies (ISS) in The Hague, in the Netherlands. She has lectured in the United States, as well as in Lebanon, Syria, and Oman. Her expertise has led her to work with the major development agencies, such as UNDP, UNICEF, and FAO. She is the author of *Dispossession and Displacement in the Modern Middle East* (Cambridge University Press, May 2010) and *Syria: The Making and Unmaking of a Refuge State* (Hurst Publishers, 2018) as well as a number of studies, including the most recent: "Refuge from Syria: Policy Recommendations" (Refugee Policy Center, Oxford, January 29, 2016).

Omar Dewachi is Associate Professor of medical anthropology at Rutgers University and cofounder of the Conflict Medicine Program at the American University of Beirut. Trained as a physician and anthropologist, Dewachi's work examines the social, medical, and environmental impacts of war on everyday life. His award-winning book, *Ungovernable Life: Mandatory Medicine and Statecraft in Iraq*, is the first study documenting the untold story of the rise of state medicine in Iraq under colonial and postcolonial regimes of rule and the consequent unmaking of state infrastructure and the exodus of medical doctors and expertise under decades of US interventions and violence in the country. His forthcoming book manuscript *When Wounds Travel* chronicles close to ten years of ethnographic research and public health practice on the social ecologies of wounds and wounding, the rise of Multi-Drug Resistant Bacteria, and the reconfigurations of health care and humanitarian geographies across the East of the Mediterranean states. He is the author of numerous publications that have appeared in a number of medical, anthropological, and global health journals, including *The Lancet*. He has worked as an advisor to organizations, such as Médecins Sans Frontières (MSF) and International Committee of the Red Cross (ICRC), on medical and humanitarian matters in the Middle East.

Neve Gordon is a professor of international law at Queen Mary University of London. Neve's research focuses on international humanitarian law, human rights, new warfare technologies, the ethics of violence, and the Israeli-Palestinian conflict. His first book, *Israel's Occupation* (University of California Press 2008), provided a structural history of Israel's mechanisms of control in the West Bank and Gaza Strip. His second book, *The Human Right to Dominate* (Oxford University Press, 2015), was written with Nicola Perugini and examines how human rights, which are generally conceived as tools for advancing emancipation, also can be used to enhance subjugation and dispossession. Most recently, he wrote with Perugini the first book on the legal and political history of human shielding. *Human Shields: A History of People in the Line of Fire* (University of California Press 2020) follows the marginal and controversial figure of the human shield over a period of

150 years in order to interrogate the laws of war and how the ethics of humane violence are produced.

Alexey Khlebnikov is a strategic risk consultant and a Middle East North Africa expert at the Russian International Affairs Council (RIAC). He works as a consultant to various entities and institutions in the United States, the Middle East, Europe, and Russia. Alexey also worked with Médecins Sans Frontières (MSF) consulting on the Middle East and Russian policy toward the region. During his Master's and PhD studies, he lived in the region working and studying in Syria, Israel, and Egypt. He has been published on international relations topics—in particular on the MENA region—in academic journals and media sources in Russia, Europe, United States, and the Middle East. He holds an MA in global public policy from the University of Minnesota, Hubert Humphrey School of Public Affairs and a BA and MA in Middle Eastern studies from Lobachevsky State University of Nizhny Novgorod. He was an Edmund Muskie fellow (2012–2014) in the United States and a research fellow at the Johns Hopkins University School of Advanced International Studies (SAIS) in 2013 and at Tel Aviv University in 2011. Alexey's research was focused on the modern transformations in the region and the Arab Uprising. Currently, he is interested in Levant, GCC, intra-Arab and intraregional tensions.

Fouad Gehad Marei is Research Associate at the University of Birmingham. His research focuses on governance, state-society relations, insurgency, and Islamist politics in the Middle East. He has research experience in Lebanon and Syria and is particularly interested in conflict dynamics and postconflict recovery. Fouad previously worked at the University of Erfurt and the Free University of Berlin in Germany and the Orient Institute in Beirut, Lebanon. He also consults for governments and think tanks on regional politics and has been involved in developing and implementing conflict stabilization and transformation programs. Fouad holds a PhD from Durham University in the United Kingdom.

Manar Marzouk is a global health researcher with a focus on health policy and health systems in refugee and conflict settings. She is currently working with the COVID-19 International Modelling Consortium (CoMo) at the University of Oxford on modeling the impact of COVID-19 mitigation measures in various regions of Syria. She is involved in several projects dealing with health systems and policy analysis in the Middle East North Africa (MENA) region. She has experience dealing with cancer care management for Syrian refugees in Jordan (WHO-EMRO, 2016), and minorities' experiences in accessing mental health services (Health

Experience Research Group, University of Oxford, 2017). Manar holds an MSc in International Health and Tropical Medicine from the University of Oxford, and a bachelor's degree in pharmacy from the University of Damascus.

Duncan McLean holds a PhD in history and is currently senior researcher with Médecins Sans Frontières for UREPH (Unité de Recherche sur les Enjeux et Pratiques Humanitaires) in Geneva. He has managed operations for MSF in both field and headquarters starting in 2002. Previously a lecturer in history at Charles University and the Anglo-American University, Prague, Duncan has also worked in policy, journalism, and history, writing and publishing in all three domains.

Hala Mkhallalati is a global public health researcher with a main focus on noncommunicable diseases, preventable interventions, and co-production. She has worked on identifying communicable-disease risk factors among women in war zone settings such as Aleppo, Syria. She also has worked on the D Magic—Diabetes in Bangladesh project while pursuing her MSc in Global Health and Development from UCL Institute for Global Health. Hala has more than five years of field experience in health policy and health systems in developing countries and conflict settings. She is a cofounder of various local public health initiatives in Syria that focus on community engagement and participation and is a founder of a local public health research team in Aleppo, Syria, where she worked in infection control and prevention for four years. Hala holds a Bachelor of Science in Pharmacy from Ebla Private University, Idlib.

Introduction

JEHAN BSEISO, MICHIEL HOFMAN,
AND JONATHAN WHITTALL

Hundreds of thousands of people have been killed and millions displaced in a decade of conflict in Syria. The devastation caused by the unrelenting war makes this crisis one of the most serious humanitarian disasters in recent history. The widely reported and available numbers— more than six million internally displaced and five million refugees, roughly half the population of the entire country—reflects only a fraction of the conflict's toll (OCHA 2019). Hundreds of thousands of people have been besieged, hospitals have been destroyed, and humanitarian access has been restricted. This has led to countless denunciations from international organizations, states, and civil society movements calling for the laws of war to be respected, sieges lifted, and humanitarian access facilitated. But beneath each of these humanitarian appeals lies a complex reality extending beyond the binary narratives that have come to define the Syria war: of an "evil regime" willing to demolish neutral hospitals in its quest to defeat a popular uprising, or of "terrorists" using hospitals to launch attacks against a legitimate government. Indeed, each reasonable demand for a more humane conduct of warfare interacts with the complexity of Syria's history and the role of social services in the postcolonial period, the evolution of the application of the law of war in the context of a war on terrorism, the lived experiences of the tactic of siege that follows Syrians across borders, the use and manipulation of humanitarian narratives to fuel complex

Jehan Bseiso, Michiel Hofman, and Jonathan Whittall, *Introduction* In: *Everybody's War.* Edited by: Jehan Bseiso, Michiel Hofman, and Jonathan Whittall, Oxford University Press. © Médecins Sans Frontières 2021. DOI: 10.1093/oso/9780197514641.003.0001 information wars, and the way in which aid delivery is both perceived by recipients and diverted by those who control its access.

This edited volume examines the politics of aid delivery in Syria by analyzing its complexities and uncovering the ways in which humanitarian aid, advocacy, and health service delivery have sometimes been complicit in a war that placed the provision, diversion, and restriction of services at the center of the battle for the Syrian state. It does this by exploring the history of health care in postcolonial state-making (Chapter 1); the fragmentation of the health system in Syria during the conflict (Chapter 2); the role of international humanitarian law (IHL) in enabling attacks on health facilities (Chapter 3); the differences between humanitarian solutions and refugee populations' expectations (Chapter 4); the way in which humanitarian actors have fed the war economy (Chapter 5); and the lived experience of siege in all its layers (Chapter 6). Finally, this volume examines how humanitarian actors have become part of the information wars that have raged throughout the past ten years (Chapter 7) and how they have chosen to position themselves in the face of grave violations of IHL (Chapter 8).

EVERYBODY'S WAR

The Syrian war started in 2011 following unarmed antigovernment protests that swept across the country in March of that year, with demonstrators demanding political and economic reforms. In Deraa, the southwestern city where the torture of children had lit the spark for the Syrian uprising, the streets were flooded with people demanding change (Macleod and Flamand 2011). As the military and police cracked down hard, these protests quickly evolved into an all-out war that has seen Syria plunged into a protracted conflict causing immeasurable human suffering. Initially, large swathes of Syria's territory were captured by armed opposition groups. Control of these territories has been wrestled back through brutal battles that have made use of large-scale airpower, besiegement, and grueling ground offensives. Whether overt or covert, foreign political, military, and operational support to parties involved in the conflict quickly became a defining characteristic of the war. The military involvement of Russia, in 2015, eventually tipped the balance in favor of the Syrian government, and the deadlock began to lift as areas under siege by Syrian forces were retaken under "reconciliation deals" often brokered by outside forces (Adleh and Favier 2017).

Although some international and regional powers rallied behind the Syrian government, a similar unity was not seen for the armed opposition.

The insurgency fragmented, some of it morphing into the notorious "Islamic State." The United States provided training, arms, and salaries to so-called moderate opposition fighters (Itani 2017). Other regional and international powers backed different parts of the divided opposition, but mostly chose to avoid a direct military engagement at the scale of that chosen by Russia and Iran. Small numbers of US and other Western troops were sent into the country, primarily to oil-producing regions to battle the Islamic State alongside forces from the Kurdish self-administration governing most of the country's east. The financial and material support of the powers backing the armed opposition groups was enough to sustain the war, but not enough to tip the scale in favor of the opposition.

The infamous slogan for many supporters of the Syrian president, Bashar al-Assad, was "Assad or we burn the country" (Al-Ghazal 2019), a symbolic phrase indicating how far people would go, on both sides of the war, to defend what they believed in.

Syria went from being a stable and peaceful host country for refugees, mainly Palestinian refugees since 1948 and also significant influxes of Iraqis following the US invasion of Iraq in 2003, to becoming a center point of regional instability that displaced millions and plunged the majority of its inhabitants into crushing poverty (Dorai 2010). In fact, in 2020, 83 percent of Syrians were living below the poverty line, and 11.7 million people were in need of humanitarian assistance—five million of whom were facing "catastrophic, critical or severe" conditions (OCHA 2019).

The level of need facing the Syrian population would suggest that Syria was somehow a neglected conflict—that the country was being ignored, out of the headlines, and off the agenda of world powers. The reality indicates the opposite: Sixteen UN Security Council resolutions have been passed on the war in Syria since 2012. An additional sixteen Security Council resolutions on Syria have been vetoed by Russia (Nichols 2020). Without a doubt, the Syrian conflict has seen unprecedented involvement of regional and global powers, including direct military interventions from four of the five permanent members of the UN Security Council—a level of international engagement not seen since the Korean War.

Syria has certainly been everybody's war. However, it has not been everybody's victory. The Syrian people have been failed. Failed by their leaders, who have besieged, starved, killed, maimed, and wounded them. Failed by their proclaimed "liberators," who used and manipulated them in endless power and territory grabs. Failed by neighboring states, which have closed their borders or offered temporary shelter in camps with poor conditions and no sustainable access to basic services. Regional powers used their geographic proximity and sectarian agendas to pour arms into the country, treating the Syrian people as pawns in a geo-strategic chess game. In a decade of war, global powers and members of the Security Council have never been able to implement a meaningful political solution and instead have sent troops, dropped bombs, and sustained the war.

HUMANITARIAN PARALYSIS

Although many nations mobilized immense financial and military power to engage in the Syrian war, the humanitarian response remained a secondary priority despite the investment made by many of the same global and regional nations that participated in the conflict. It is not unfair to say that humanitarian organizations were paralyzed in responding sufficiently to the needs generated by the conflict. This book explores some of the humanitarian consequences that came to define the war in Syria, including the fragmentation of the health system (Chapter 2), attacks on hospitals (Chapter 3), the refugee crisis (Chapter 4), and the role of siege as a tactic (Chapter 6). The abysmal humanitarian response to each of these needs represented yet another failure for the Syrian people.

Humanitarian aid delivery became quickly entangled into the polarized sides of the Syria war. The Syrian government sought to control aid delivery from Damascus, placing heavy restrictions on United Nations agencies, the International Committee of the Red Cross, and the few other international agencies permitted to work, often preventing them from freely crossing front lines to reach the most vulnerable. Other organizations unable to work in Syria officially, together with civil society groups associated with the uprising and organizations set up by the Syrian diaspora, began delivering aid across neighboring borders into territory controlled by the armed opposition without permission from the Syrian government. Aid was quickly stained with the political divisions and colors of the conflict; organizations crossing the border were considered "pro-opposition," while those working from Damascus were seen as "pro-regime."

For Médecins sans Frontières (MSF), this was no different. From the start of the deterioration of the situation in Syria, MSF asked to work officially from Damascus. The organization aimed to work with the authorization of the Syrian government to reach communities based on their needs. But access was never granted. Faced with this obstacle, MSF adapted and began providing assistance across the border from neighboring countries in response to rising needs. By 2013, MSF was running six hospitals in opposition-controlled areas of Syria. "We had to repeatedly negotiate agreements with different local commanders to ensure respect for our presence, for the safety of our teams, and for non-interference with our medical activities," Dr. Joanne Liu, then the international president of MSF, wrote in 2015. "The groups changed frequently, and we renegotiated agreements with commanders from Jeish el Mujahideen, Islamic Front, Jahbat Al Nusra, different factions of the Free Syrian Army, and ISIS (later renamed Islamic State—IS), among others" (Liu 2015). Yet in January 2014, ISIS abducted thirteen MSF staff members, eight of whom were released within hours, and five of whom were held for five months. Following the incident, MSF withdrew the majority of its teams from Syria and resorted to providing distant support to networks of Syrian medics working in areas in need (Liu 2015). When the tactic of siege became a core feature of the Syrian war, humanitarian actors working from Damascus as well as from across the borders were unable to assist the hundreds of thousands of people who were trapped out of reach.

THE LIMITS OF MEDICAL HUMANITARIAN SOLIDARITY

In March 2018, MSF released an open letter to the doctors under siege in Eastern Ghouta stating that "we were confronted again with the limits of our ability to provide you and your facilities with assistance when the needs were highest" (Bilbao 2018). Dr. Amani Ballour, who has written the foreword to this book, was one of those doctors to whom this open letter was addressed. Dr. Ballour, a pediatrician working in an underground hospital in the besieged enclave of East Ghouta, describes the harrowing reality of the massacres she witnessed, including a chemical attack. She recalls how she woke up in the middle of the night to find hundreds of corpses, people who had suffocated without wounds or blood, many of them children. A UN investigation team visited the site some days after the attack and found "clear and convincing evidence" of the use of the nerve agent Sarin, delivered through surface-to-surface rockets (United Nations 2013). For Dr. Ballour, it was clear this was yet another crime committed by the Syrian government. The resulting disarmament, in which the Syrian government was stripped of its chemical weapons, "confiscated the weapon, but they left the criminal on the loose." For Dr. Ballour, the hollow condemnations from the so-called international community throughout the suffocating siege could not match the horrors faced by even one child in East Ghouta.

While humanitarian organizations, including MSF, drew attention to the consequences of such sieges, they also contributed to a framing of the crisis through a humanitarian lens only, a convenient distraction for those who could deliver a political solution. Ultimately, Dr. Ballour and her colleagues were left to deal with the enduring consequences on their own.

The MSF letter to the doctors of East Ghouta, written toward the end of the siege, went on to state that "at this very moment, our ability to assist in providing healthcare in East Ghouta is almost non-existent." The stark contrast between the cries for help from doctors inside Eastern Ghouta and the paralysis of an emergency medical organization like MSF is a clear illustration of an aid system helpless in the face of large-scale suffering.

Below the surface of this failure in aid response, however, lies a deeper reality shaped by multiple factors explored through the chapters of this book.

HUMANITARIAN POLITICS

Humanitarian organizations repeatedly appealed to the responsibilities of the warring parties to facilitate humanitarian assistance in Syria (Parker 2013, 3–5). Implicit in this appeal was the claim by humanitarian organizations to a form of neutrality in the Syrian war. This appeal, however, was ultimately incompatible with the way in which the Syrian state and the opposition saw aid delivery—both its provision and its denial—as part of the battle for statehood, a reality outlined in Chapter 1 of this book, "Contested Statehood: The Politics of Health Care in Syria." Those providing services to areas controlled by the opposition were seen by the Syrian government as complicit in directly challenging the legitimacy of the state, through their taking over essential services that the state had considered within its exclusive remit since its postcolonial establishment. In the same logic, opposition groups co-opted humanitarian assistance to enforce their own legitimacy to the population, as they were led by people shaped by the same era in which medical care and, in their case, contesting the legitimacy of the state, were inextricably linked.

In the eyes of the Syrian state, humanitarian actors such as MSF were far from neutral. This was only compounded and reinforced by public statements made by MSF calling for the recognition of the de facto partitioning of the Syrian state in the delivery of assistance. Such calls were more a partisan war cry than an appeal for impartial aid delivery when put in the context of the history of health care in Syria. Indeed, in Chapter 1 of this book, Omar Dewachi, Fouad Gehad Marei, and Jonathan Whittall outline how the history of health care in Syria has shaped the way in which wartime health care has been delivered and controlled.

Chapter 2, by Manar Marzouk, Hala Mkhallalati, and Aula Abbara, takes the analysis of the politics of health care further by exploring the way in which health care fragmented during the civil war. The Chapter examines how at least four health systems have emerged as a result of various geopolitical, fiscal, and humanitarian drivers. Chapter 2, "Health System Fragmentation and the Syrian Conflict," makes the case for increased collaboration between the various fragments of the Syrian health system.

Within the context of such politicized healthcare delivery, however, the appeals made by organizations such as MSF to the warring parties to respect the protection of health facilities under international humanitarian law (IHL) may have missed an important evolution that Neve Gordon explores in Chapter 3. These appeals overlooked the way in which IHL itself may have been facilitating attacks on health facilities in Syria. In his chapter, Gordon explores how the dominant way of understanding attacks on health care was through the lens of IHL, and how the primary way to seek accountability was through legal redress. Gordon exposes, however, the disconnect between the law, which requires the neutrality of independent health professionals, and the way in which local health actors understood their role in the Syrian war.

The humanitarian norm that appeals to the protection of healthcare provision is based on the separation between war-makers and health providers. Yet, as Gordon points out, "this separation is extremely difficult to sustain due to the function of health care and the particular role of health professionals in the war effort." Both the Syrian government and health workers themselves consider their role to be partisan. For the Syrian government, this is due to the way health care was seen as part of the postcolonial state-building project, as outlined by Dewachi and colleagues in Chapter 1. For health workers, as Gordon shows, the provision of health care under fire was part of the resistance effort.

The convergence of war and health, combined with the way in which the law "offers medical units protections only to assert the primacy of national laws and their ability to annul the protections," has allowed for an environment of unhindered violence directed toward health workers. And yet the law has remained a primary recourse for advocacy against attacks on health workers.

Dewachi and colleagues appeal for a re-politicization of the understanding of health in conflict, and Gordon argues for a complete ban on hospital bombings, which would accommodate the reality of health being provided as part of political efforts. This would ensure that these health actors, providing essential—albeit highly politicized—services, would not fall through the cracks of exemptions found in IHL.

While attacks on hospitals continued unabated in the Syrian war, the numbers of displaced continued to rise. Refugees crossing the borders into neighboring countries exposed another way in which there was a discrepancy between the reality on the ground and the standardized approaches taken by humanitarian actors. Dawn Chatty, in Chapter 4, argues that it was in Turkey—where the humanitarian presence was limited, and the Turkish state and civil society took the lead without the support of the UNHCR in responding to refugee needs—that the refugee response was provided "without undermining refugee agency and dignity." In other contexts, Chatty points out that "global templates for humanitarian assistance built from experiences in very different contexts and among populations of significantly different makeup are not easily integrated into Middle Eastern concepts of refuge, hospitality, and charity."

Chatty criticizes the "architecture of assistance" that was "built upon templates developed over the past few decades largely among agrarian and poor developing countries." She concludes that "without a serious effort to make humanitarian 'solutions' fit the context of the Middle East, success will continue to be muted, at best, and damaging, at worst."

While Chatty demonstrates the way in which humanitarian actors were slow to adapt to the aspirations of regional refugees, Duncan McLean, in Chapter 5, presents an example of how humanitarian aid did adapt to the realities of the Syria war, and the context of besiegement in particular, by reaching populations under siege through utilizing the corruption mechanisms of informal networks and smugglers. In this case, however, it was through humanitarian actors' adaptations to the realities of besiegement that the aid system contributed to the war economy.

Although healthcare provision has been a deeply political process steeped in the dynamics of the Syria conflict, the reality is that humanitarian aid also was provided by states as a substitute for meaningful foreign policy. The cruel irony is that the provision of this aid, "in the place of any collective will to address either the root causes or extreme violence," has arguably contributed to the prolongation of the conflict through its contribution to a war economy. McLean describes a process of aid delivery so intertwined with the endemic corruption of the war as a business model that it generated a form of "entrepreneurial neutrality" in the sense that businesses, entrepreneurs, and all warring parties worked together in profiting from the system.

What McLean ultimately shows is that while aid was given as a substitute for meaningful foreign policy, it also played a role in fueling a war economy that sustained the efforts of the belligerents who were so protected by international political failures.

The complicity in the suffering in Syria extended beyond the complex war economy of which humanitarian actors formed an integral part. In Chapter 6, Jonathan Whittall, one of the editors of this volume, explores the way in which siege follows civilians from within Syria to the places they seek refuge. Whittall argues that "political opponents otherwise separated by interests and ideologies appear united in their use of siege tactics. There is a chain of complicity, in generating human suffering and exploiting it, from Syria to its neighbors and from Europe to its international allies." He adds that humanitarian actors, whether within Syria or in neighboring countries, are at worst contributing to sustaining besiegement and at best diverting attention from the political choices that lie behind the various forms of containment.

The endless siege experienced by Syrians raises questions as to whether these humanitarian failures were technocratic shortcomings or rather the inevitable consequence of a long chain of complicity and profiteering among states that produced refugees, hosted them, and funded the responses to their needs. Humanitarian actors implemented programs in a policy environment that sought to contain—to endlessly besiege—Syrians, rather than to assist them in finding protection. In her research, Chatty found that protection, not resettlement, is what the majority of Syrians aspire to. The inability and unwillingness of states to provide this protection, Chatty argues, is a stark contrast to the solution for temporary protection that Europe was able to find, when it had the political will to do so, for 1.2 million Bosnians during the war of 1992 to 1995.

HUMANITARIAN POSITIONING

Within a context where aid delivery is part of the battle for the state, and where complicity in the suffering of Syrians extends from humanitarian actors to regional and international powers, the credibility of the humanitarian narrative comes under great scrutiny.

Alexey Khlebnikov, in Chapter 7, describes his concern with the "one-sided" nature of humanitarian actors' narratives from Syria, promoted by international NGOs through their large presence in the media. Khlebnikov believes that this "contributed heavily to the growing alienation and intransigence between the opposition and the government, making any meaningful dialogue between them nearly impossible." According to Khlebnikov, humanitarian actors, including MSF, contributed to the spread of disinformation in the Syria war due to their presence on only one side of the conflict, which he argues requires a heavier regulation of humanitarian work in the future.

However, humanitarian actors such as MSF continued to defy the constraints on providing assistance by finding ways to deliver aid inside areas under siege and by speaking out against the complete disregard for civilian life and infrastructure by the warring parties. The politics of this war, and the role of aid at the center of it, were, however, ultimately far bigger than MSF. The organization failed to turn the tide against the attacks on hospitals through its approach of naming and shaming the perpetrators of hospital bombings, as explored by Michiel Hofman, another editor of this volume, in Chapter 8. This was possibly due to the way in which IHL is wired to provide exemption for warring parties, as outlined by Gordon, or because of MSF's failure to deliver consistent messages necessary to generate popular pressure on offending nations, as argued by Hofman.

Khlebnikov's casting of the state in the role of the primary regulator of humanitarian aid was ultimately what happened in the Syria war. The Syrian government's denying assistance to the population and disrespecting the laws of war, while absorbing the denunciations that followed such actions, centered the state as both perpetrator and aid responder. Whether through checkpoints, sieges, raids, and bombing campaigns on the one hand, or through the control of supplies of medicine, food, and aid on the other, the result was the same: The Syrian state was always in control. For a state seemingly so unphased by public opinion, the focus on its ability to deny and allow access to services arguably only served to amplify its control and project its sovereignty. In this way, the Syrian state centered its own sovereign control by being the focus of diplomatic efforts to ensure humanitarian access. At the same time, the attacks on service delivery allowed the Syrian government to limit its opponents' ability to gain legitimacy from the delivery of services that could have posed a credible alternative to the state.

DIVERSE PERSPECTIVES ON A SHARED FAILURE

Although the response of humanitarian actors did not match the immensity of the Syrian population's needs, most organizations' ways of working on the ground played into the polarization of aid delivery. For organizations such as MSF, through its attempt to circumvent restrictions on aid, its much-needed delivery of assistance has arguably contributed to fueling a war economy. In neighboring countries, the approach to aid delivery has proved to be far removed from what refugees themselves see as the needed role of humanitarian action.

Meanwhile, humanitarian needs and the response to those needs have taken center stage on diplomatic platforms, often in place of meaningful foreign policy. What the collection of perspectives in this edited volume suggest, however, is that focusing on the consequences of the war, rather than on its causes, has been a victory for the sovereignty of the Syrian state. Through the humanitarian lens, with its focus on the need for access, and the outcries at the appalling attacks on health facilities, the Syrian state remained the uncontested and only legitimate actor in both the maintenance and destruction of the infrastructure of life in Syria. Meanwhile, states from neighboring countries all the way to Europe prolonged the siege on Syrians through the implementation of policies that denied Syrian civilians access to safety and assistance.

A humanitarian complicity has characterized the politics of aid delivery in the Syrian war. Organizations such as MSF inconsistently named and shamed perpetrators of the violations of international humanitarian law, allowing the Syrian and Russian governments to easily discredit these claims to their own support base and to reinforce their position that humanitarians were part of the contestation of Syrian statehood.

In Syria, a "humanitarian war" of a different kind was fought. Instead of Western states exerting their hard power under the guise of humanitarian concern (as seen in the wars in Iraq or Libya), or trying to win hearts and minds through the delivery of humanitarian aid (as seen in Afghanistan and Iraq), humanitarian aid delivery in Syria became the battleground itself, the battleground on which the future for the Syrian state was fought.

Within such a context, aid actors crossed borders, supplied opposition networks, denounced the government, and called for more aid to opposition areas: All of this was never seen by the warring parties as a form of independent humanitarian concern for the people of Syria, but rather as a battle cry for the overthrow of the Syrian state.

No single perspective can capture all the nuances of the Syrian war. A defining feature has been the way in which information, particularly that coming from humanitarian actors, has been used and misused to promote various agendas. This edited volume examines the politics of aid in "everybody's war" from as many different perspectives as possible: those of researchers in the United Kingdom and Russia; those of the broader Middle East region; those of medical practitioners, including one who has herself experienced siege in Syria; and those of aid practitioners who have encountered the dilemmas and witnessed the war's devastation.

This book is edited by MSF staff, and the various chapters often draw extensively on MSF material made available to researchers. The book also presents the perspective of a number of MSF staff members who have worked on the Syria war for the past decade, including the editors themselves. But this book does not provide an "MSF view" on the Syrian war—partly because no such homogenous view exists within the organization, and partly because this is not a story about one humanitarian organization, but rather about the broader complexities of aid delivery in one of the defining conflicts of the twenty-first century.

Ultimately, each chapter provides a piece of a puzzle demonstrating humanitarian complicity in the Syrian war. This book is the story of the complex politics of aid in everybody's war.

REFERENCES

Adleh, Fadi, and Agnes Favier. 2017. *"Local Reconciliation Agreements" in Syria: A Non-Starter for Peacebuilding.* Middle East Directions. June 2017. https://cadmus.eui.eu/bitstream/handle/1814/46864/RSCAS_MED_RR_2017_01.pdf?sequence=1.

Al-Ghazal, Zaki Kaf. 2019. "The Syrian Regime's Slogan 'Assad or We Burn the Country' Must Not Become Reality." *Middle East Monitor*, May 21, 2019. https://www.middleeastmonitor.com/20190521-the-syrian-regimes-slogan-assad-or-we-burn-the-country-must-not-become-reality/.

Bilbao, Lorena. 2018. "Letter to the Doctors of East Ghouta." Médecins sans Frontières, March 28, 2018. https://www.msf.org/syria-letter-doctors-east-ghouta.

Dorai, Mohammed Kamel. 2010. "Palestinian and Iraqi Refugees and Urban Change in Lebanon and Syria." Middle East Institute, April 19, 2010. https://www.mei.edu/publications/palestinian-and-iraqi-refugees-and-urban-change-lebanon-and-syria.

Itani, Faysal. 2017. "The End of American Support for Syrian Rebels Was Inevitable." *Atlantic*, July 21, 2017. https://www.theatlantic.com/international/archive/2017/07/trump-syria-assad-rebels-putin-cia/534540/.

Liu, Joanne. 2015. "Unacceptable Humanitarian Failure." Médecins sans Frontières, March 11, 2015. https://www.msf.org/syria-unacceptable-humanitarian-failure.

Macleod, Hugh, and Annasofie Flamand. 2011. "Tortured and Killed: Hamza al-Khateeb, Age 13." Al Jazeera, May 31, 2011. https://www.aljazeera.com/features/2011/05/31/tortured-and-killed-hamza-al-khateeb-age-13/.

Nichols, Michelle. 2020. "Russia, China Veto Syria Aid via Turkey for Second Time This Week." Reuters, July 10, 2020. https://www.reuters.com/article/us-syria-security-un-idUSKBN24B2NW.

OCHA (Office for the Coordination of Humanitarian Affairs). 2019. *2019 Humanitarian Needs Overview: Syrian Arab Republic.* OCHA, March 2019. https://hno-syria.org/#resources.

Parker, Ben. 2013. "Humanitarianism Besieged." *Humanitarian Exchange* 59 (November 2013): 3–5. https://odihpn.org/magazine/humanitarianism-besieged/.

United Nations. 2013. *Report of the United Nations Mission to Investigate Allegations of the Use of Chemical Weapons in the Syrian Arab Republic on the Alleged Use of Weapons in the Ghouta Area of Damascus on 21 August 2013,* September 16, 2013. http://undocs.org/A/67/997.

CHAPTER 1
Contested Statehood

The Politics of Health Care in Syria

OMAR DEWACHI, FOUAD GEHAD MAREI, AND
JONATHAN WHITTALL

In February 2012, in its first public position on the unfolding armed conflict in Syria, Médecins Sans Frontières (MSF) published a series of testimonies gathered from Syrian doctors working in the country. The testimonies described the challenges and horrors facing doctors trying to treat wounded patients and protesters injured by Syrian authorities (MSF 2012). In its report, MSF denounced the use of "medicine as a weapon of persecution" in Syria and called on the government to "re-establish the neutrality of healthcare facilities" (MSF 2012). In a press release published a year later, MSF further decried that aid was not being distributed "equally" between government- and opposition-controlled areas and argued that "areas under government control receive nearly all international aid, while opposition-held zones receive only a tiny share" (MSF 2013). In an opinion piece, two MSF staff members criticized humanitarian actors working with the authorization of the Syrian government and called on those aid agencies to recognize "the de-facto partitioning of the state" (Weissman and Rodrigue 2013).

Such calls from humanitarian actors, which on other occasions claimed neutrality, played into the polarization of the Syrian conflict. The Syrian government actively controlled aid delivery and distribution from Damascus, with the support of Russia and Iran. Aid from Damascus was distributed by

Omar Dewachi, Fouad Gehad Marei, and Jonathan Whittall, *Contested Statehood* In: *Everybody's War*. Edited by: Jehan Bseiso, Michiel Hofman, and Jonathan Whittall, Oxford University Press. © Médecins Sans Frontières 2021. DOI: 10.1093/oso/9780197514641.003.0002 the United Nations, the Syrian Arab Red Crescent society, and a handful of other organizations working in government-controlled areas. Meanwhile, aid was delivered across the borders from neighboring countries by opposition groups, civil society activists, and Western humanitarian actors.

While the Syrian government sought to defend itself through the maintenance of its prerogatives to deny or provide social services, the opposition sought to contest the state and its legitimacy through the provision of its own services and ultimately through the creation of an alternative infrastructure of healthcare delivery. The de facto partitioning of the country according to the delivery of services was in fact the fault line for the battle over the future of the state.

As the conflict progressed, innumerable attacks targeted healthcare facilities and medical personnel (Fouad et al. 2017). The destruction of healthcare facilities has left health services decimated, with an estimated 782 medical personnel killed during the first five years of the conflict, among whom 32 percent were doctors (Omar 2020, 200). Moreover, already by 2012, over 50 percent of the country's hospitals and clinics were deemed to be functioning at low or no capacity due to lack of staff, equipment, or medicine, or due to irreparable damage to facilities (Kherallah et al. 2012). By 2015, several facilities operated at less than 1 percent functionality (Omar 2020, 199).

The widely used public health narrative to describe the dynamics of the Syrian war has often centered on the blockages of humanitarian aid by the Syrian government and its violation of international humanitarian law (IHL) through attacks on hospitals, which are intended to undermine the opposition. This has highlighted the centrality of health care to the politics of the conflict, while at the same time portraying health as a neutral subject of war and politics. We suggest that such a framing fails to acknowledge a more nuanced historical and sociological understanding of healthcare politics and its entanglement in the histories and practices of statecraft in Syria. The politics of health in Syria rendered humanitarian aid delivery a threat to Syria's sovereignty. This is because in Syria, as in other postcolonial nation-states, the delivery of social services has been an important component of establishing and maintaining state control, a control central to the government's claim of sovereignty.

Furthermore, such accusations assume that the politicization and the "weaponization" of health care during the conflict is a one-sided undertaking. While we neither excuse nor defend attacks on health providers and humanitarian aid workers and facilities, we contend that the contemporary humanitarian system, with the majority of funding coming from states and international organizations in opposition to the Syrian government, should not be depoliticized or decontextualized as being entirely benevolent, neutral, and nonpartisan. Beyond the obvious humanitarian needs, opposition groups and those sympathetic to their cause instrumentalized the provision of health as part of their bid to replace the state and delegitimize the government.

In the analysis that follows, we provide a historical overview of the relationship between health care and state-making in Syria. Although this is not intended to be an entirely comprehensive overview, we outline some of the major social, political, economic, and environmental transformations that have shaped state power in Syria and the region. Based on this history we reflect on the limits of technocratic and public health discourses of the conflict and demonstrate how health care and humanitarian relief became a contested battleground of Syrian statehood.

THE STATE OF MEDICINE IN SYRIA

It is critical to situate health care in Syria within a genealogy of state-building, to better understand its dismantlement under contemporary conditions of war. Although Syria has been governed by an authoritarian one-party system, the governance of the country has extended beyond state policing, Ba'ath Party ideologies, coercion, and violence. Over the past decades, Syria also has been governed through the rapid development of the country's healthcare system and its material and human infrastructures. The building and maintenance of public hospitals, the development of a pharmaceutical industry, the devising of vaccination campaigns, and the training and equipping of the country's medical professionals were central to securing the social and political legitimacy of the state in Syria. In other words, the state's control over the Syrian population involved not only oppressive modes of government, but also the provision of social welfare, including health and health care—what we refer to as productive modes of power. Although not mutually exclusive, both coercive and productive modes of power shape how social behavior is regulated, underpin the state's claim to legitimacy and sovereignty, cultivate a sense of citizenship and belonging, and redefine relations between state and society. Historians of Syria and the Middle East have examined the politics of health and its transformation under colonial and postcolonial projects, highlighting the central role of medical organizations and the responses to public health events (such as epidemics) in understanding the workings of state power and the shaping of state-society relations (Blecher 2002; Dewachi 2017; Longuenesse et al. 2012; Neep 2012). Such historical and anthropological framing understands health and health care as part of broader fields of social life, such as education, welfare, family, and economy—all of which became central to the state-making and social-engineering projects of colonial and postcolonial Syria. Thus, understanding the role of health care in Syria prior to and during the conflict requires a closer look at the history of state medicine and public health over the past century.

Since the mid-nineteenth century, the Syrian province, which included present-day Lebanon, assumed an important role in the production of healthcare infrastructure across the Middle Eastern region. Starting in the 1860s, Ottoman authorities in Syria developed expansive urban health practices. Municipalities began to carry out the collection of waste, the inspection of restaurants and abattoirs, and the policing of beggars, with increasing emphasis on the moral responsibility of individual citizens to adopt health and hygiene strategies. The historian Daniel Neep argues that these urban health strategies allowed the Ottoman authorities to use biopolitical techniques to govern the local population, thereby shaping the formation of the modern political subject in Ottoman Syria (Neep 2012).[1] Moreover, the training of locals in modern Western medicine expanded with the inauguration of missionary medical schools (both American Protestant and French Catholic) in the city of Beirut, in modern-day Lebanon, and with the further development of Ottoman medical schools concerned with the training of the local Arab populations in the Arabic-speaking provinces of the Ottoman Empire (Tibawi 1966; Blecher 2002). Graduates of these medical schools hailed mostly from elite local families. They occupied central positions in Ottoman public health administration, as well as in the expansion of medical services to the local Arab populations. The training of local doctors was seen as an important strategy of "rule and control"; it contributed to the growth of the Ottoman state and was part of an attempt to win the support of an ambivalent local population (Blecher 2002).

After the fall of the Ottoman Empire and the establishment of the French mandate over the Syrian province (1920–1946), the expansion of medicine and public health became linked to France's efforts to create a nation-state and modernize everyday life (Neep 2012). Medicine and public health held a special place in the Mandatory project, as it became part of France's "civilizing" mission, *Mission civilisatrice*, as well as a central strategy in the development of institutions regulating population dwelling and mobility. Medical and public health organization further shaped practices of the local communities through the engineering of urban space and its connections to the rural peripheries (Neep 2012; Blecher 2002).

Health and education continued to be linked to the agendas of political elites following Syrian independence in 1946 (Longuenesse et al. 2012).

The postmandate period witnessed major political upheavals and military coups, resulting in numerous rewritings of the constitution. Consistently, and in line with many decolonizing ideologies in the global South at the time, health and education became two major symbols of modernization, development, and the forwarding of a socially progressive agenda (Longuenesse et al. 2012). Syrian authorities presented health and education as a right for all in line with other socialist and quasi-socialist state-building projects in the region, such as in Egypt and Iraq (Dewachi 2017). During this period, economic growth was based on the availability of agricultural land for cultivation, mostly financed by the country's rich mercantile urban classes (WHO 2006). But despite the ambitious "health for all" discourse, rural and peripheral areas continued to suffer from a lack of access to, and availability of, resources and services. At the same time, such discourse often was marred by the ruling elites' multitude of political, social, and economic interests. Despite the geographical disparities, Syria witnessed rapid improvements in development and health indicators throughout the mid-twentieth century.

In 1963, the Ba'ath Party came to power through a military coup. Hafez al-Assad's ascent to the presidency in 1971 consolidated Ba'ath party control over Syria. Government policies considered the shortfalls of previous governments, especially in terms of the marginalization of the Syrian peripheries. In fact, the Ba'ath leadership from the military establishment, including the president, hailed from just such a rural background—a class pattern that shaped the dynamics of their ascent to power in the country (Batatu 1999). The government's policies viewed the expansion of health and education in the underdeveloped areas of rural Syria as a means to reach out to broader segments of the population, thus expanding the state's reach beyond the urban centers and consolidating the Ba'ath Party's control countrywide. Moreover, the state embraced large-scale development projects to expand industry, agriculture, and infrastructure. The government introduced land reforms and nationalized the country's major industries and foreign investments, as the state assumed greater control over centralized economic decision-making, planning, and the regulation of commercial transactions. Despite these social and economic investments in the agricultural sector, the country witnessed major demographic shifts in terms of continuous migration from the rural countryside to the booming cities. Between 1960 and 1970, Syria's urban population increased from 50 percent to 57 percent of the total population, as the country's economy shifted from a predominantly agrarian one to an economy based on services and commerce (WHO 2006).

Investment in health care was reflected in the country's health and development indicators in the decades after the Ba'ath Party assumed control. According to data from the Syrian Ministry of Health, over close to four decades (1970–2009), life expectancy at birth increased from 56 years to 73.1 years, infant mortality decreased from 132 per 1,000 live births to 17.9 per 1,000, and under-five mortality dropped dramatically, from 164 to 21.4 per 1,000 live births (Kherallah et al. 2012). During the same period, maternal mortality also fell significantly, from 482 to 52 per 100,000 live births. But these indicators concealed wide social and economic discrepancies between urban centers and the countryside, a fact that would continue to shape the state-building project in Syria in the years leading to the conflict in 2011 (Kherallah et al. 2012).

During the decades of Ba'ath Party reign, medical education occupied a central stage in the development of the state and was instrumentalized for achieving multiple objectives. First, it allowed poor rural individuals to access education and join the ranks of the urban medical-class professionals, thus ensuring a mode of state socialization and upward social mobility. Second, it provided an exclusionary measure for those whose loyalty to the ruling elite was in question, and it offered an incentive to join party ranks as a form of access to medical education. Third, the state's investments in training health professionals and expanding the country's healthcare infrastructure positioned Syria as a major hub for training of medical doctors and expertise, and put Syria on a fast track for development, given that many health and social indicators improved dramatically during this period. Fourth, it allowed Syria's movement toward self-sufficiency, as the state invested in supporting a national and affordable pharmaceutical industry to address the increasing demands for therapeutics in the country and the region.

It is important to mention that the pharmaceutical industry in Syria grew from eleven manufacturers in 1970 to fifty-four in 2005, 82 percent of which belonged to the public sector. In 2005, Syria produced about forty-six hundred drugs, which covered around 90 percent of the country's needs, and it was exporting to forty-two different countries (WHO 2006). Moreover, during the same period, the state increased its number of medical schools and intake of medical students, and thus the number of Syrian doctors able to cover the population's needs. Yet even with a significant increase in the number of doctors, Syria continued to lag behind, especially in light of the country's rapid population growth and the increasing need for primary health care, partly due to the emigration of Syrian medical professionals. In fact, immigrant Syrian physicians played an important role in the development of healthcare systems in the oil-rich countries of the Gulf Cooperation Council (GCC) and helped high-income countries in northern and western Europe overcome their prevailing shortage of medical specialists.[2] As in other regional states, many doctors in Syria were reluctant to serve in the public sector, favoring the private sector for its better financial prospects.

HEALTH CARE IN THE ERA OF ECONOMIC LIBERALIZATION

In 2006, the World Health Organization (WHO) published a report examining the state of Syria's health system in light of the country's liberalization reforms (WHO 2006). The report provided a historical overview of Syria's progress in terms of improving health indicators and commended the Syrian government for implementing major market and bureaucratic reforms. It also offered new directions for liberalizing the health system. Unfortunately, WHO public health reporting failed to account for the complex, long-term effects of Syria's marketization and other liberalizing interventions on population health in the social and economic sectors. In fact, the impact of economic liberalization policies during the decades leading to the Syrian civil war fomented crony capitalism—an economic system featuring strong relationships between business leaders and government officials—and "undermined even the semblance of equality and productivity in the Syrian economy in favour of the few" (Haddad 2011, xiii–xiv). This new political economy was instrumental in shaping the roots of the conflict (Abboud 2015; Daher 2020).

Syria embarked on economic liberalization in the early 1990s, following the country's fiscal crisis in 1986. The adoption of "economic pluralism" (*al-ta'adudiyya al-iqtisadiyya*) as a national economic policy in 1991 acknowledged the role of the private sector alongside the public sector. The private sector's share of the country's gross fixed capital formation rose from 30 percent in 1975 to 50 percent in 1987, and to 66 percent in 1992 (Hinnebusch 1995, 318).

The Syrian government's turn toward economic liberalization accelerated in the 2000s, after Bashar al-Assad succeeded his father, Hafiz al-Assad. Having consolidated his power, Bashar al-Assad announced in 2005 his government's adoption of a Social Market Economy (Seifan 2011), the first "official and public expression in the four decades [of Ba'ath Party rule] of a desire to move away from a state-centred economy and toward a mixed economy" (Haddad 2011, 4). This allowed the country to attract foreign direct investments from the GCC, as well as to appease Western powers and lessen the international pressure on Damascus. This economic opening capitalized on the fortunes accumulated by Syrian expatriates who benefited from preferential employment opportunities in the oil-rich GCC monarchies. The flow of remittances underpinned a growing private sector that was expanding to fill in gaps left by a retreating public sector. This resulted in the reintroduction of the bourgeoisie and of foreign business interests in the political sphere as "partners" in the nexus of political and economic power (Abboud 2015).

Politically, this resulted in a rearrangement within the ruling party and the political establishment. Entrenching the patrimonial nature of the Syrian state, sections of the old guard and state and public-sector strongmen were replaced with officially sanctioned business moguls and relatives of Bashar al-Assad (Haddad 2011, xv; Daher 2020, 58). Meanwhile, the networks of private-sector tycoons loyal to the president replaced the Ba'ath Party as the main vehicle for political mobilization and patronage, and substituted the corporatist organizations of the Ba'athist regime (such as trade unions and workers' associations) as the mechanisms of sociopolitical organization (Daher 2020, 35, 75).

Although gradual and piecemeal, the deleterious outcome of Syria's neoliberal reforms came at the expense of Syrian society. Government spending as a proportion of GDP dropped from 48 percent in 1980 to only 25 percent in 1997 (Goulden 2011, 192); the labor participation rate dropped from 52 percent in 2001 to 42 percent in 2010;[3] and inequality soared, with 5 percent of society controlling an estimated 50 percent of national income in 1997 (Perthes 2004, 10), while poverty rates reached 14.3 percent in the same year (Matar 2016, 109).

Liberalization measures also resulted in inflation and rising prices. This was accompanied by austerity measures, including the diminution of the state's vast subsidy system and the abandonment of state-sanctioned price ceilings in favor of marketization, affecting the prices of key food items, gas and fuel, and housing (Abboud 2015, 55). As a consequence, large segments of the Syrian middle class were pushed into poverty and driven to join the urban subaltern in the sprawling urban slums, where rural migrants fleeing draught and economic inopportunity in the countryside lived in informal housing, estimated to be as high as 40 percent of total housing in the urban peripheries (Ismail 2013; Abboud 2015).

Thus, as Bassam Haddad (2011, xiv) notes, "the reservoir of discontent in Syria" on the eve of the popular uprising in 2011 ran "much deeper than one might think on the basis of the modest number of protesters we have witnessed."

The Syrian transformation from a command economy—an economy in which production, investment, prices, and incomes are determined by the central government—to crony capitalism took place within the context of global transformations and geopolitical realignments after the Cold

War. The period's dramatic changes ushered in a new era of global health politics, characterized by the introduction of neoliberal interventions to reform public sectors, including health care, across the world. The logic and discourse of the "structural adjustments" prescribed by major international financial organizations (IFOs) and imposed by Western economies since the mid-1980s called on governments—especially in the global South—to privatize the productive sectors of national economies and outsource the provision of social welfare. These interventions transformed healthcare systems globally, especially through the re-entrenchment of the state from its social responsibilities—thus increasing inequalities and inequities across the globe (Kim et al. 2002). The shrinking of the state due to economic liberalization policies allowed for the emergence of a plethora of nonstate actors to which some of the state's *de jure* prerogatives were relegated, including the use of force, justice, law enforcement, and social welfare provision.

Despite the Syrian government's turn to economic liberalization, however, the state retained, to an impressive degree, its control over the legitimate use of force as well as the provision of population welfare. For example, in contrast to other Middle Eastern countries, in Syria communal forms of justice and arbitration remained minimal, whereas the state's tight grip on national resources and the prerogative to manage population and welfare shifted from the state-party-military to the state-business elite. This is not to say that the Syrian state did not embark on, or at least entertain, the desire to slowly hand over some of its stately prerogatives to a burgeoning sector of nonstate (albeit co-opted and heavily regulated) charitable and community-based associations. But for much of Bashar Al-Assad's reign, health care and other welfare-provision sectors did not promise private-sector or foreign investors the easy-come, easy-go investment returns desired (Marzouq 2011; 2013).

This limited liberalization of social welfare in Syria was not the result of market rationale alone; it was also a strategic decision of the Syrian state to retain its control over population welfare. In other words, while the Syrian government selectively and partially conceded its monopoly by allowing the emergence of private-sector services (Marzouq 2013, 49–50), the Syrian state retained its overall control of the provision of education and health care, even as the quality and quantity of public-sector health services diminished (Daher 2020, 94).

For instance, the Syrian government allowed the expansion of an Islamic charitable sector, sanctioned and controlled by the state. This sector mobilized Muslim preachers, Islamist intellectuals and public figures, religiously motivated entrepreneurs, and a network of faith-based charities. The rise of the Islamic charitable sector accelerated in the 1990s, as the Syrian government sought to strengthen its relations to the Sunni majority (Daher 2020, 54). But the expansion of this sector was kept in check not only by the watchful gaze of the state and its security apparatus (as is the case in much of the Arab world), but also by the Syrian state's ability to retain its claim over population welfare. For example, although the first recorded license granted to an Islamic movement to establish an elementary school dates to the 1970s (Imady 2016, 73), Islamic charities associated with the state-sanctioned "moderate" Islamist milieu were only rarely granted licenses to operate faith-based schools, hospitals, or clinics (Khatib 2011; Pierret 2013). This is in stark contrast to, for instance, Egypt and Jordan, where an expansive network of faith-based schools, hospitals, and clinics stepped in to substitute the state following its decision to out-source welfare provision in line with the prescriptions of international financial institutions (Clark 2003).

Concomitant with this turn to economic liberalization, a steady rift emerged between those who held the view that health care is an essential constituent of the state's claim to legitimacy and proponents of more radical economic liberalization. For the former, the state's exclusive claim over the tools of population management—healthcare provision, education, justice, and security—ensured the government's ability to mitigate the effects of economic liberalization and lessen their costs for aggrieved population groups, thus ensuring regime stability. For proponents of radical liberalization, the state's reluctance to extend the maxims of community and private-sector leadership from the business to the welfare sectors resulted in their eventual parting with the Syrian government and its social market economy.

On the eve of the Syrian uprising, health and healthcare infrastructure occupied a central position at the heart of the Syrian government's claims to legitimacy and sovereignty, although it already was being challenged by the economic liberalization reforms. Indeed, as the country approached the outbreak of civil unrest in March 2011, the government slowed its promarketization reforms and austerity measures, and demonstrated signs of "a reversion to more public-sector friendly policies" (Haddad 2011, xiii), exemplified, for example, by the elimination of the hitherto pivotal post of deputy prime minister for economic affairs, occupied until March 2011 by Abdallah Al-Dardari.[4] As popular protests broke out in Syria in March 2011 and the country slowly descended into civil war, the politics of health would become a pivotal point of contention and a battleground between the Syrian government and civilian and armed opposition groups.

The Syrian conflict emanated from a popular uprising whose people demanded greater freedoms, voiced grievances against the state's policies, and expressed deep discontent with the practices of the state's coercive apparatuses. This was motivated, in part, by similar uprisings in Egypt, Libya, and Tunisia—a wave of protest that came to be known as the "Arab Spring." The popular mobilizations demanded regime change and voiced discontent with police brutality and widening socioeconomic cleavages. Although this may be true of the initial mobilizations of early 2011, the Syrian uprising quickly took on a life, or several lives, of its own.

The trajectory of these mobilizations is rooted in and influenced by contextual factors including, but not limited to, socioeconomic realities on the ground, regional and global power relations, and a litany of social tensions. This was exacerbated by the rapid armament of antigovernment factions, the intervention of regional and global powers, the rise of an opposition in exile, and the Syrian government's brutal response to popular demands. Together, these resulted in the gradual militarization of the Syrian uprising and the country's descent into a protracted conflict—a dynamic that can no longer be reduced to the limits of its initial roots as a popular uprising. Advertently or inadvertently, the abundance of political, military, and humanitarian support for the various belligerents of the Syrian war—provided by actors as varied as the United States, Russia, Iran, Turkey, Saudi Arabia, and international organizations and humanitarian nongovernmental organizations (NGOs)—contributed to the protraction of the conflict.

At the start of the Syrian uprising in 2011, reports emerged of wounded protesters being arrested and healthcare providers being targeted by state security forces for providing treatment to the wounded. In 2012, the Syrian government passed a law that healthcare and humanitarian assistance not approved by the state was illegal and could be seen as support to terrorism (Human Rights Council 2013). This forced most healthcare structures providing care to the injured to go underground (Gladstone and Browne 2019). These informal, makeshift health facilities themselves were targeted by the state. Hospitals repeatedly came under attack, which in turn increased the fear of both providing and receiving health care. While Western donors and regional powers sought to find ways of channelling assistance to communities cut off from services, in line with their interests, the Syrian government's restrictions on aid delivery set the limits on the provision of humanitarian assistance outside its jurisdiction. As the conflict in Syria escalated, the government response became characterized by siege tactics, indiscriminate bombing, and mass displacement.

When it comes to understanding the unravelling of the healthcare system in the context of the Syrian conflict, terms such as "government-controlled" and "rebel-controlled" areas simplify and obscure the complex realities on the ground. At the early stages of the uprising, opposition activists established Local Coordination Committees (LCCs) in response to the contraction of government control. LCCs morphed into Local Councils (LCs), which assumed responsibility for the provision of public services, such as health and education, maintenance of the legal system, law and order, and attention to administrative and bureaucratic affairs in areas beyond the control of the government. As the scholar Samer Abboud rightly notes, however, this "has not led to the growth of alternative or coherent state institutions but rather to a patchwork of administrative authorities that are backed up by violent networks" (Abboud 2015, 248).[5] Moreover, he describes the relationship between this "patchwork of administrative authorities" and the "patchwork of armed brigades" constituting the armed opposition as one of "fluidity and the constant shifting of alliances."

On the other hand, the boundary between the government and the opposition was more fluid than is often acknowledged. For example, the government remained the main provider of health care to the majority of Syrians living inside the country despite the contraction of its territorial control between 2012 and 2015. According to several civilian opposition activists who spoke to one of us (Marei) in the period between 2012 and 2014,[6] government agents and civil servants continued to receive their salaries and instructions from Damascus, even in areas controlled by armed opposition groups.[7] Much of this provision of services was carried out through the maintenance of facilities with the help of middlemen, as well as through the regular payment of salaries to civil servants and government employees in nongovernment-controlled areas.

Interestingly, evidence on the ground suggested that the continued provision of government services in nongovernment-controlled areas did not always undermine the role of LCs and civilian and armed opposition groups. For instance, a civilian member of the opposition LC in the town of Mahaja (Daraa province) explained to one of us (Marei) that even in March 2013—one year after the town had come under opposition control—local government agencies performed their duties, and employees continued to receive instructions and salaries from Damascus via intermediaries. He added that "government agencies and the LC worked together," noting that "since civil servants of the governments are natives of Mahaja, a teacher or a physician often worked for both government and opposition schools and clinics . . . or at least they cooperated and coordinated with their colleagues, friends, and relatives who worked [on the other side of the government/opposition divide]."[8] The vice president of the LC in the border town of Al-Bou Kamal (Dayr Al-Zor province) corroborated this, saying that "government employs relatives, friends, and neighbours of ours. . . . We oppose the regime, but we are keen that [government agencies] continue to perform their jobs and serve the people. . . . This lessens the burden on [the LC] and the governing councils of the civilian opposition."[9] An internal MSF report also noted that routine vaccination programs were being carried out in Ghouta and Homs by the Ministry of Health, even in so-called opposition-controlled clinics.

Meanwhile, the fragmentation of the healthcare system in Syria, the dangers physicians faced, and the economic and career incentives abroad resulted in a mass exodus of Syrian doctors, with as many as half the country's thirty thousand physicians leaving Syria by the end of 2015 (Omar 2020, 200). Instead, other providers of health care in Syria included NGOs, diaspora-founded organizations, and nongovernmental networks of medical practitioners. MSF, for example, provided assistance through hands-on medical projects in areas under the control of the armed opposition, which was where access could be negotiated. Aid providers also supported makeshift hospitals and medical networks where direct access for the organization was not possible, including in areas besieged by government forces.

The provision of health outside state channels has been considered a direct threat to the Syrian government's claim to legitimacy and the prerogatives of the state. As such, government forces have repeatedly targeted the healthcare-provision capabilities of opposition factions, their foreign backers, and humanitarian aid actors operating across national borders without the authorization of the Syrian state. Indeed, the government in Damascus has consistently viewed humanitarian aid provided in areas beyond its control by organizations claiming impartiality and neutrality as a partial and direct act of support to the armed opposition. For instance, the Syrian ambassador to the United Nations, Bashar Ja'afari, told the United Nations Security Council in 2018 that "like the Islamic State," MSF was behaving like "terrorists without borders."[10]

The Syrian government's approach to controlling the provision of services as a core part of the defense of its fragmenting sovereignty has been enabled by the same logic as the global "war on terror"—which ironically has often labeled Syria as a terrorist state. This approach obscures the distinction between civilians and combatants, resulting in large swaths of population in areas under control of the armed opposition being treated as terrorists or enablers of terrorism, and therefore considered by the Syrian state and its allies as legitimate targets.

The Syrian government's framing of humanitarian aid and social-service provision as a threat to its legitimacy and sovereignty, through the creation of parallel governance that challenges its own legitimacy, goes a long way toward explaining government strategies during the Syrian conflict. For example, besiegement has played a tactical role in the war,[11] often tied to contestation over the delivery of public welfare functions deemed prerogatives of the state. Although the reasons for the use of the tactic of siege are numerous, it is relevant to note that several of the areas that suffered heavy and prolonged besiegement during the Syrian war were the urban peripheries that mushroomed following Bashar al-Assad's liberalization reforms after 2000. These peripheries saw the Syrian state struggle to manage health—among other core welfare services—as one of the main pillars of its claim over statehood and population management. The current war has seen the further erosion of the government's claim to statehood over these urban peripheries. Controlling these zones of limited state control through the denial of the essentials for life—and then reclaiming them—can be understood as an assertion of the monopoly the state seeks to hold over population welfare as a way to defend its statehood.

THE PITFALLS OF DECONTEXTUALIZATION

The understanding of the politics surrounding aid response and its shortcomings in Syria has often been reduced to the simple dichotomy of the "evil regime" versus "the opposition," with civilians—"the victims"—caught in the middle. Moreover, much of the literature relating to the Syrian war and its health implications focuses on the brutal attacks against health facilities and health workers. According to Annie Sparrow, the "Assad regime has come to view doctors as dangerous, their ability to heal rebel fighters and civilians in rebel-held areas a weapon against the government" (Sparrow 2013). Similarly, a *Lancet* article published in 2017 argued that the conflict in Syria presented new and unprecedented challenges that undermined the principles and practices of medical neutrality in armed conflict; it called for a response to the systematic violations of international humanitarian law. Other research points to the use of indicators monitoring attacks on healthcare facilities as a way to "add granularity to traditional indicators of violence (e.g., such as civilian casualties) to develop a more nuanced understanding of the warring tactics used and violence against civilians in the Syrian conflict" (Ri et al. 2019).

The legal stance of this work is understandable. However, such arguments often overlook the role of historical and sociological processes in shaping the politics of health. As the provision of health has been shaped by the politics of statecraft in colonial and postcolonial Syria, attacks on health care are not unique to the Syrian conflict. The blurring of health care and warfare had become ripe across the region with the unfolding of the US-led "war on terror" in Iraq, Afghanistan, and Pakistan, as well as in Gaza, Palestine (Dewachi 2015). Such decontextualized approaches to framing and analyzing the Syrian conflict are echoed in the often highly bureaucratic and diplomatic workings of international and intergovernmental organizations operating in the humanitarian field. For example, the secretary-general of the United Nations established several Boards of Inquiry (BoI) charged with investigating "incidents" involving or resulting in the destruction or damage of schools, hospitals and healthcare facilities, displacement centers, and other civilian objects as a result of military operations.[12] Several of these civilian targets were placed on a "deconfliction list" established by the United Nations to help facilitate their protection in the context of the Syrian war. According to the documents made public by these BoIs, belligerents in the Syrian war compromised the safety of "the courageous humanitarian workers who risk their lives every day to help those who are most in need in the midst of conflict" (United Nations 2016). The BoI reports considered the impact of hostilities on civilian and humanitarian sites in northwestern Syria "a clear reminder of the importance for all parties to the conflict to observe and ensure respect for international humanitarian law," reiterating that "any measures that Member States may take . . . must be consistent with their obligations under international law, in particular international humanitarian law, international human rights law and international refugee law" (United Nations 2020).

Although it is undoubtedly necessary and essential to appeal to the Syrian government to cease attacks against hospitals and medical facilities, doing so alone overlooks the underlying dynamics of conflict and its entanglements in health and healthcare politics. Health in conflict cannot be understood as a technical problem defined by depoliticized models and indicators. This technocratic approach to conflict management reproduces misleading binaries between "courageous humanitarian workers" (United Nations 2016) and violators of international law—binaries that ultimately undermine the ability of healthcare practitioners and humanitarian organizations to navigate the politics of war effectively. It also inadvertently entrenches the role of health actors as active protagonists in the contestation over the Syrian state.

Indeed, the tally sheets of IHL violations are much needed to high-light the repetitive nature and scale of attacks on healthcare workers and infrastructures in Syria. Having said this, the calls for "medical neutrality" seem to flatten the long political history of health and health care in the logics and practices of state-making across the region, as well as the complexities of health politics that shape practices of various state and nonstate actors involved in conflict and humanitarian relief. Moreover, defining health care as a "weapon of war," and its destruction as a "weapon of mass destruction," obscures the deeper political meanings and processes of health care that have shaped, and continue to shape, the struggles over the legitimacy of the state in Syria.

REPOLITICIZATION OF HEALTH

Healthcare delivery has never been a neutral business in Syria. Thus, it is crucial to repoliticize the understanding of health in the context of the Syrian conflict, wherein its providers are not simply neutral in their delivery of health care or victims of IHL violations but are also part of an active battle for the future of the state.

A more political, contextual analysis of the relationship between healthcare provision on the one hand, and the state's claim to sovereignty and legitimacy on the other, offers an explanation for the Syrian government's hostility toward humanitarian and health workers, and for the ferocity of its attacks on healthcare facilities operating outside its jurisdiction. Embattled in its monopoly over the use of force, the Syrian government continues to fight, viciously, for its control over the management of life and death of the populace. Civilian and armed opposition groups alike organize and seek support in providing health care and other means of subsistence and population management in opposition-controlled areas, where they present themselves to the Syrian people as alternative providers of health care. In so doing, they challenge the Syrian government's monopoly over violence, as well as its claim to being the sole or main provider of health.

Though attacks on hospitals violate the prescriptions of IHL and the laws of armed conflict, it should not be surprising that field and state-run hospitals, clinics, and rapid-response medical teams and supplies became a target for government forces and opposition groups. Although neutrality and impartiality are frequently invoked by intergovernmental and international humanitarian organizations to protect health and aid workers under IHL, such claims are often unhelpful in the context of the Syrian conflict. This is because humanitarian organizations operating outside the jurisdiction of the Syrian government have contributed to the delegitimization of the embattled Syrian state and provided legitimacy to the state-making aspirations of the Syrian opposition. The government's suspicion is further exacerbated by the fact that major humanitarian and aid organizations operating in Syria are tightly linked to or funded by Western states hostile to the Syrian government.

As the war in Syria enters a new phase characterized by the postwar political economies of reconstruction, health in postconflict Syria will most likely remain a highly disputed field of competing interventions and narratives, with national and international, state and nonstate actors competing over stakes in public health. Those who succeed in delivering this service will have an upper hand in the contestation for the future of the Syrian state.

NOTES

1. This is not unique to Ottoman Syria. Historians of nineteenth-century Egypt have argued that while the spread of modern medicine and education to the population at large had immeasurable modernizing potentiality, it also provided the Egyptian state with new tools of "modern governmentality" to control and survey populations and bodies in turn-of-the-century Egypt. See, for example, Hatem (1997) and Fahmy (1998). Similarly, Ebrahimnejad (2010) suggests that attempts to modernize medicine and medical education in nineteenth-century Iran were integral to the centralization of power and the expansion of the military—in short, the advent of the modern nation-state.
2. For example, on Germany, see Loss et al. (2020).
3. See data from the World Bank: https://data.worldbank.org/indicator/SL.TLF.CACT.NE.ZS?locations=SY.
4. As Deputy Prime Minister for Economic Affairs (2005–2011) and Minister of Planning (2006–2008), Abdallah Al-Dardari played a pivotal role in shaping the promarket agenda that defined economic policy in Syria starting in 2005. Al-Dardari was dismissed from his position in March 2011. In September of the same year, he joined the United Nations Economic and Social Commission for Western Asia (ESCWA), first as director of the Economic Development and Globalization Division and then, starting in 2014, as deputy executive secretary of ESCWA. In 2012, he oversaw the establishment of the National Agenda for the Future of Syria (NAFS), an initiative intended as a platform for "technical dialogue for Syrian experts from different backgrounds to talk about reconciliation and peacebuilding in post-conflict Syria" (see https://nafsprogramme.info/about-nafs/who-we-are.html). Al-Dardari is accused of maintaining ambiguous relationships with the Syrian government, diasporic business groups and networks, and civilian and armed opposition groups.
5. This is perhaps with the exception of the areas controlled by the Islamic State between 2014 and 2018, where the jihadi proto-state embarked on establishing institutions, hierarchical structures, and bureaucracies with a state-like semblance.

6. Based on interviews and focus group discussions with civilian opposition activists and members of LCCs and LCs in Damascus and seven other governorates. Interviews were conducted by Fouad Gehad Marei between 2012 and 2014 as part of a series of studies on civilian opposition structures in nongovernment-controlled areas in Syria.
7. This corroborates a similar claim made by the Syrian Ministry of Health.
8. Interview (March 2013; Istanbul, Turkey). Interviewee anonymized to guarantee his security. Interview was conducted by Fouad Gehad Marei as part of a series of studies on civilian opposition structures in nongovernment-controlled areas in the Syrian conflict.
9. Interview (April 2013; Istanbul, Turkey). Interviewee anonymized to guarantee their security. Interview was conducted by Fouad Gehad Marei as part of a series of studies on civilian opposition structures in nongovernment-controlled areas in the Syrian conflict.
10. See the comments from Bashar Ja'afari at https://www.un.org/press/en/2018/sc13302.doc.htm.
11. See Chapter 6 in this volume by Whittall.
12. For example, UN Secretary-General Ban Ki-Moon established in October 2016 a Board of Inquiry to investigate the targeting of a UN-Syrian Arab Red Crescent humanitarian convoy in Urum al Kubra (Big Orem), near the city of Aleppo, Syria, on September 19, 2016. In August 2019, Ki-Moon's successor, Secretary-General António Guterres, established the Board of Inquiry into attacks on civilian targets in northwestern Syria following the signing of the Memorandum on Stabilization of the Situation in the Idlib De-escalation Area by the Russian Federation and Turkey in September 2018.

REFERENCES

Abboud, Samer N. 2015. *Syria*. Malden, MA: Polity Press.
Batatu, Hanna. 1999. *Syria's Peasantry, the Descendants of its Lesser Rural Notables, and their Politics*. Princeton, NJ: Princeton University Press.
Blecher, Robert I. 2002. "The Medicalization of Sovereignty: Medicine, Public Health, and Political Authority in Syria, 1861–1936." PhD thesis, Stanford University.
Clark, Janine A. 2003. *Islam, Charity, and Activism: Middle-Class Networks and Social Welfare in Egypt, Jordan, and Yemen*. Bloomington: Indiana University Press.
Daher, Joseph. 2020. *Syria after the Uprisings: The Political Economy of State Resilience*. London: Pluto Press.
Dewachi, Omar. 2015. "Blurred Lines: Warfare and Health Care." *Medicine Anthropology Theory* 2 (2). https://doi.org/10.17157/mat.2.2.185.
Dewachi, Omar. 2017. *Ungovernable Life: Mandatory Medicine and Statecraft in Iraq*. Stanford, CA: Stanford University Press.
Ebrahimnejad, Hormoz. 2010. "Glimpses of Relationship Between Hospital, State and Medicine in Nineteenth-Century Iran." In *Perilous Modernity: History of Medicine in the Ottoman Empire and the Middle East from the 19th Century Onwards*, edited by Anne Marie Moulin and Yeşim Işıl Ülman, 97–103. Istanbul: ISIS Press Istanbul.
Fahmy, Khaled. 1998. "Women, Medicine, and Power in Nineteenth-Century Egypt." In *Remaking Women: Feminism and Modernity in the Middle East*, edited by Lila Abu Lughod, 35–72. Princeton, NJ: Princeton University Press.

Fouad M. Fouad, Annie Sparrow, Ahmad Tarakji, Mohamad Alameddine, Fadi El-Jardali, Adam P Coutts, Nour El Arnaout, Lama Bou Karroum, Mohammed Jawad, Sophie Roborgh, Aula Abbara, Fadi Alhalabi, Ibrahim AlMasri, Samer Jabbour. 2017. "Health Workers and the Weaponisation of Health Care in Syria: A Preliminary Inquiry for *The Lancet*–American University of Beirut Commission on Syria." *The Lancet Health Policy* 390 (10111): 2516–26. https://doi.org/10.1016/S0140-6736(17)30741-9.

Gladstone, Rick, and Malachy Browne. 2019. "In Syria, Health Workers Risk Becoming 'Enemies of the State.'" *New York Times*, December 4, 2019. https://www.nytimes.com/2019/12/04/world/middleeast/syria-health-workers-persecution.html.

Goulden, Robert. 2011. "Housing, Inequality, and Economic Change in Syria." *British Journal of Middle Eastern Studies* 38 (2): 187–202.

Haddad, Bassam. 2011. *Business Networks in Syria: The Political Economy of Authoritarian Resilience*. Stanford, CA: Stanford University Press.

Hatem, Mervat F. 1997. "The Professionalization of Health and the Control of Women's Bodies as Modern Governmentalities in Nineteenth-Century Egypt." In *Women in the Ottoman Empire: Middle Eastern Women in the Early Modern Era*, edited by Madeline C. Zilfi, 66–80. Leiden: Brill.

Hinnebusch, Raymond A. 1995. "The Political Economy of Economic Liberalization in Syria." *International Journal of Middle East Studies* 27 (3): 305–20.

Human Rights Council. 2013. *Assault on Medical Care in Syria*. Human Rights Council, Twenty-Fourth Session, Agenda Item 4, September 13, 2013.

Imady, Omar. 2016. "Organisationally Secular: Damascene Islamist Movements and the Syrian Uprising." *Syria Studies* 8 (1): 66–91.

Ismail, Salwa. 2013. "Urban Subalterns in the Arab Revolutions: Cairo and Damascus in Comparative Perspective." *Comparative Studies in Society and History* 55 (4): 865–94.

Khatib, Line. 2011. *Islamic Revivalism in Syria: The Rise and Fall of Ba'thist Secularism*. London: Routledge.

Kherallah, Mazen, Tayeb Alahfez, Zaher Sahloul, Khaldoun Dia Eddin, and Ghyath Jamil. 2012. "Healthcare in Syria Before and During the Crisis." *Avicenna Journal of Medicine* 2 (3): 51–53.

Kim, Jim Yong, Joyce V. Millen, Alec Irwin, and John Gershman, Eds. 2002. *Dying for Growth: Global Inequality and the Health of the Poor*. Monroe, ME: Common Courage Press.

Longuenesse, Elisabeth, Sylvia Chiffoleau, Nabil Kronfol, and Omar Dewachi. 2012. "Public Health, the Medical Profession, and State Building: A Historical Perspective." In *Public Health in the Arab World*, edited by Jabbour, Samer, Giacaman, Rita, Khawaja, Marwan, and Nuwayhid, Iman, 7–20. Cambridge: Cambridge University Press.

Loss, Julika, Yamen Aldoughle, Alexandra Sauter, and Julia von Sommoggy. 2020. "'Wait and Wait, That Is the Only Thing They Can Say': A Qualitative Study Exploring Experiences of Immigrated Syrian Doctors Applying for Medical License in Germany." *BMC Health Services Research* 20: 342. https://doi.org/10.1186/s12913-020-05209-2.

Marzouq, Nabil. 2011. "The Economic Origins of Syria's Uprising." *Al-Akhbar English* (online).

Marzouq, Nabil. 2013. "Al-tanmîyya al-mafqûda fî sûrîyya." In *Khalfîyyât al-thawra al-sûrîyya: Dirâsât sûrîyya*, edited by Azmy Bishara, 35–70. Doha: Arab Center for Research and Policy Studies.

Matar, Linda. 2016. *The Political Economy of Investment in Syria*. London: Palgrave Macmillan.

MSF (Médecins Sans Frontières). 2012. "Medicine as a Weapon of Persecution." MSF, February 8, 2012. https://www.msf.org/syria-medicine-used-weapon-persecution.

MSF (Médecins Sans Frontières). 2013. "MSF Criticises Aid Imbalances." MSF, news release, January 29, 2013. https://www.msf.org/syria-msf-criticises-aid-imbalances.

Neep, Daniel. 2012. *Occupying Syria Under the French Mandate: Insurgency, Space and State Formation*. Cambridge: Cambridge University Press.

Omar, Abdulaziz. 2020. "Understanding and Preventing Attacks on Health Facilities During Armed Conflict in Syria." *Risk Management and Healthcare Policy* 13: 191–203. https://doi.org/10.2147/RMHP.S237256.

Perthes, Volker. 2004. *Syria Under Bashar Al-Assad: Modernisation and the Limits of Change*. London: Oxford University Press and Routledge.

Pierret, Thomas. 2013. *Religion and State in Syria: The Sunni Ulama from Coup to Revolution*. Cambridge: Cambridge University Press.

Ri, Sayaka, Alden H. Blair, Chang Jun Kim, and Rohini J. Haar. 2019. "Attacks on Healthcare Facilities as an Indicator of Violence Against Civilians in Syria: An Exploratory Analysis of Open-Source Data." *PLOS ONE* 14 (6). https://doi.org/10.1371/journal.pone.0217905.

Seifan, Samir. 2011. *The Road to Economic Reform in Syria*. Fife, Scotland: University of St. Andrews Centre for Syrian Studies.

Sparrow, Annie. 2013. "Syria's Assault on Doctors." *New York Review of Books*, November 3, 2013. https://www.nybooks.com/daily/2013/11/03/syria-assault-doctors/.

Tibawi, A. L. 1966. *American Interests in Syria 1800–1901*. Oxford: Clarendon Press.

United Nations. 2016. "Letter from the Secretary-General to the President of the Security Council," December 21, 2016. https://digitallibrary.un.org/record/853646?ln=en.

United Nations. 2020. "Letter from the Secretary-General to the President of the Security Council," April 6, 2020. https://digitallibrary.un.org/record/3856791?ln=en.

Weissman, Fabrice, and Marie-Noëlle Rodrigue. 2013. "Syria: Breaking the De Facto Humanitarian Embargo against Rebel-Held Areas." Centre de Réflexion sur l'Action et les Savoirs Humanitaires, March 19, 2013. https://www.msf-crash.org/en/publications/war-and-humanitarianism/syria-breaking-de-facto-humanitarian-embargo-against-rebel.

WHO (World Health Organization). 2006. *Health System Profile: Syria*. http://digicollection.org/hss/documents/s17311e/s17311e.pdf.

CHAPTER 2

Health System Fragmentation and the Syrian Conflict

AULA ABBARA, MANAR MARZOUK,
AND HALA MKHALLALATI

Syria's health system has been devastated by a protracted conflict that has left it politicized and fragmented, with multiple subnational health systems functioning within the country's borders. The preconflict health system was centralized and increasingly privatized, with a heavy emphasis on specialist or hospitalist care. The postconflict health system has faced multiple insults, which have exacerbated preconflict poor governance and inequalities; in addition, the gap between people living in urban and rural areas has widened, as it has among people who can and cannot afford out-of-pocket healthcare payments.

Since the onset of conflict, at least four health systems have emerged as a result of various geopolitical, fiscal, and humanitarian drivers. As we approach almost ten years of conflict, the main subnational health systems are: areas under the control of the Syrian government, which account for two thirds of the country and are under the remit of the Ministry of Health; areas in the northeast, which are under the Autonomous Administration of North and East Syria and include Al-Hasakah, Raqqa, Deir Ezzor, and parts of the Aleppo governorate; northwest Syria, which is under opposition control and includes the northern Idlib governorate, as well as parts of Aleppo and the northwest Hama governorate; and an 8,835-square-kilometer area of the northern Aleppo governorate along the Turkish border, which is under Turkish control, where services are provided by the Turkish Ministry of

Aula Abbara, Manar Marzouk, and Hala Mkhallalati, *Health System Fragmentation and the Syrian Conflict* In: *Everybody's War*. Edited by: Jehan Bseiso, Michiel Hofman, and Jonathan Whittall, Oxford University Press. © Médecins Sans Frontières 2021. DOI: 10.1093/oso/9780197514641.003.0003

Health. These subnational health systems differ in regard to funding, governance, key stakeholders, models of health-service delivery, and degrees of destruction to health facilities and related infrastructures. These health systems have also evolved over time—in some instances geographically, in other instances due to changes in the level of conflict, funding, and the closure of borders for cross-border humanitarian aid. In this chapter, we explore the evolution of the four subnational health systems and factors influencing the delivery of health care across the country, and we use the COVID-19 pandemic as a lens to highlight crucial challenges for all these systems.

BACKGROUND

Syria's conflict has devastated its health system, which has come under strain due to attacks, the forced exodus of healthcare workers, and the increasing health needs of Syria's population. Deliberate attacks on healthcare facilities have left at least 50 percent of them nonfunctional (Omar 2020). This is expected to result in short- and long-term consequences for the health system and the health of the Syrian population. The destruction has occurred alongside the population's changing needs: chronic diseases have gone undiagnosed or been poorly managed; the rate of communicable disease has increased; and disabilities and mental health complaints have risen. Although the conflict has affected different geographical regions to different extents, arguably all areas have been either directly or indirectly affected by the conflict.

The escalation to violence in Syria occurred after peaceful uprisings against the government, which began in March 2011, were brutally suppressed (Fouad et al. 2017). As the conflict became more protracted, all aspects of the health system needed to transition from an initial emergency response to a longer-term response, particularly in areas outside government control. By mid-2012, opposition forces had captured rural areas in the north, east, and south of the country, and they eventually were able to capture urban areas including parts of Damascus and Aleppo. As the conflict has progressed and the Syrian government has taken back territory—leaving, as of 2020, only areas in the northeast and the northwest outside its control—it has become increasingly evident that multiple health systems now exist within Syria's borders. Each has its own governance structures, funding streams, and stakeholders, and each faces different challenges. This has become increasingly evident as the COVID-19 pandemic has spread across the region, affecting the areas differently and inspiring disparate responses.

The four subnational health systems have evolved as a result of various conflict-related, humanitarian, financial, and geopolitical influences, resulting in different governance, leadership, and organizational and health system structures. Institutions and facilities outside areas under the control of the Syrian government have been left with a power vacuum of unrecognized universities and independent initiatives affecting the training and accreditation of healthcare workers (Bdaiwi et al. 2020). There is little communication or collaboration across these health systems—a risk to the population's future health. This lack of cooperation already has contributed to outbreaks of communicable diseases—for example, a polio outbreak in northeast Syria in 2017–2018 (WHO 2020c)—and has led to challenges coordinating the COVID-19 pandemic, which has exposed existing fractures within the health system and overwhelmed health-system capacity across all areas.

A FRAGMENTED AND POLITICIZED HEALTHCARE SYSTEM

Before the conflict, Syria's health system already had become increasingly privatized, with more emphasis on specialist and hospital-based care and an underdeveloped primary healthcare system (Kherallah et al. 2012). Poor leadership from the Ministry of Health alongside poor governance had led to geographical inequalities, with more emphasis on urban compared with rural areas (Abbara et al. 2015; Kherallah et al. 2012). This contributed to a mismatch between available services and the population's needs, with services and healthcare workers more concentrated in the larger cities of Damascus, Aleppo, and Homs without needed services. Public health initiatives also were underdeveloped, with few effective population measures—such as smoking cessation programs—enforced. With regard to the health of the population, Syria already had been facing an epidemiological transition from communicable to noncommunicable diseases with high rates of hypertension, diabetes, and smoking-related illnesses. These preexisting factors affected how the existing health system was able to respond to conflict.

The postconflict health system is fragmented into multiple subnational health systems (Abbara et al. 2020). For example, attacks on health care have disproportionately affected areas outside Syrian government control (Fouad et al. 2017). Yet the health of the population across the country has been adversely affected by the conflict, which has contributed to an economic crisis with high unemployment (estimated at 43 percent of those of working age in 2019 (Syrian Arab Republic UN Country Team 2020), though that figure has likely risen to 50 percent due to COVID-19), inflation, and limited access to essentials such as food and fuel, with around 80 percent of the population estimated to be subsisting below the poverty line (St. Andrews University 2017). As a result, the health system has become increasingly politicized, often along sectarian lines, with secondary consequences on the health of the population. The COVID-19 pandemic has further strained the health system and negatively contributed to the attritions to the health of the population; in addition, it has exaggerated inequities (Abbara et al. 2020).

The conflict also has affected the social, development, education, and economic sectors, which has only magnified the negative effects of the conflict, the COVID-19 pandemic, and regional contributing factors, such as the effect of the economic collapse in Lebanon on the Syrian economy. Then there are the effects of violence, with the destruction of health and relevant infrastructures resulting in direct and indirect impacts on the population. As of March 2020, it was estimated that there had been 348,000 to 586,000 deaths caused directly by violence (Syrian Observatory for Human Rights 2020), though estimates vary widely depending on methodology and accuracy of recording (Mowafi and Leaning 2018). In 2014, the United Nations declared it was almost impossible to get reliable deaths numbers in Syria (Specia 2018). In 2017 Guha-Sapir and colleagues analyzed data from the Violations Documentation Center in Syria between March 2011 and December 2016, noting 143,630 conflict-associated deaths that had sufficient data for analysis (Guha-Sapir et al. 2018). Of these, 71 percent were civilian deaths, with shelling and air bombardments responsible for 57 percent of them. Violence was responsible for 74 percent of civilian-women deaths and 70 percent of civilian-children deaths (Guha-Sapir et al. 2018). These numbers do not take into account the indirect deaths caused by the conflict, as a result of limited access to health care, medication, and vaccinations, and as a consequence of malnutrition and poverty.

EVOLUTION OF THE SUBNATIONAL HEALTHCARE SYSTEMS

The subnational health systems have evolved within different microcontexts and influences, and have been differentially affected by violence, displacement, funding, and international support. They have different characteristics and structures, which influence how they deliver care to the populations they serve. Some of the health systems are more studied than others, allowing greater understanding of how they have evolved, how governance has evolved, and how the subnational health system can be strengthened.

In areas under Syrian government control, the health system is more privatized, with a greater emphasis on secondary or tertiary care and an underdeveloped public or primary healthcare system; this is similar to how Syria's health system was structured before the conflict (Kherallah et al. 2012). Access to services in this area is inequitable due to accusations of interference with health and humanitarian aid; the health system tends to favor populations loyal to the Syrian government and to exclude populations in retaken areas, such as Dera'a in the south (Chatham House 2019). The health system in northwest Syria has been heavily influenced by the presence of local and international nongovernmental organizations (NGOs), many of which provide cross-border humanitarian aid via Turkey; this is coordinated by the World Health Organization-led Health Cluster, based in Gaziantep, in Turkey. Though the humanitarian health response to needs has been fragmented and significantly underfunded, promising initiatives have emphasized primary health care, midwifery training, and mental health programs. Areas under Turkish control share health services and structures aligned to the Turkish national model of health care; this system has been the least explored in public health literature. As before the conflict, northeast Syria remains under-resourced in terms of funding and healthcare services. This area of the country has its own governance authority; it maintains relations with areas under Syrian government control to help in accessing health care and humanitarian aid, though this access is impeded by bureaucracy and local authorities' interference with aid (Human Rights Watch 2020a). The following map shows the various regions of control (see Figure 2.1).

The United Nations (UN) Office for the Coordination of Humanitarian Affairs established a "Whole of Syria" approach in 2014, seeking to coordinate the humanitarian responses to the Syrian conflict from Turkey, Jordan, and Syria (Damascus) using the 2015 Syrian Strategic Response Plan. In September 2016, however, more than eighty aid groups, including the main Syrian humanitarian organizations from the Whole of Syria aid strategy, withdrew due to allegations that the United Nations and the Syrian Arab Red Crescent (which has close ties to the Syrian government) were allowing the state to interfere with the delivery of humanitarian aid, which was not equitably delivered to areas in need (Chatham House 2019).

Another important influence on the delivery of humanitarian aid across Syria is UN Security Council Resolutions on cross-border aid. Because of the Syrian government's influence on the provision of humanitarian aid across the country, the UN Security Council in 2014 passed Resolution 2165, which authorized humanitarian aid to enter Syria and be delivered to areas outside state control through four border crossings (OCHA 2020c),

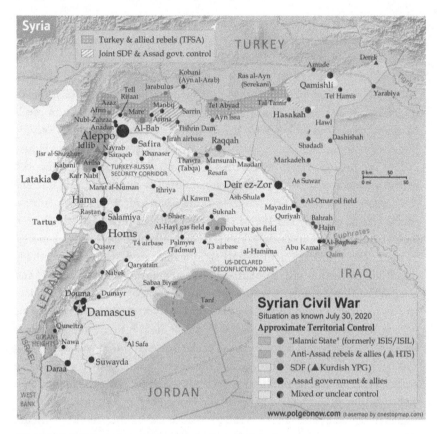

Figure 2.1. This map shows the various regions of control.
Source: "Syria Control Map & Report: Frontlines Stable—July 2020." 2020. Political Geography Now. https://www.polgeonow.com/2020/07/syria-controlled-areas-map-2020.html.

bypassing Damascus. This resolution faced annual renewal. In January 2020 a partial renewal only (and for only six months) was passed, resulting in the closure of the Yarubieh crossing on the Syria–Iraq border, which had previously allowed humanitarian aid to the northeast (Human Rights Watch 2020a); and the closure of the Ramtha crossing on the Syria–Jordan border, which had allowed aid delivery to southern Syria, but to areas now retaken by the Syrian government. This partial renewal was a result of a veto threat by the Russian and Chinese governments. In July 2020, the Bab Al Salam crossing to northwest Syria was closed, leaving only the Bab Al Hawa crossing to the northwest open. These changes have affected the COVID-19 response and the ways in which the health systems in northwest and northeast Syria can respond to the health and humanitarian needs in affected regions. Areas in the northeast of Syria have been placed at a particular disadvantage, as bureaucracy and interference with aid have hampered the flow of humanitarian assistance from Damascus (Human Rights Watch 2020a). If the resolution keeping the Bab Al Hawa crossing to the northwest open is not renewed in July 2021, this could be catastrophic for the three to four million people in the northwest who rely on this crossing for aid, because cross-line aid from areas under Syrian government control is almost nonexistent due to ongoing hostilities.

CENTRALIZED AND SPECIALIZED: THE HEALTH SYSTEM IN AREAS UNDER SYRIAN GOVERNMENT CONTROL

Though the areas under Syrian government control (other than retaken areas) have been among the least affected by direct violence, they have been severely affected by economic crisis (including knock-on effects of the economic collapse in Lebanon), interrupted supply chains, and insufficient resources. In areas under Syrian government control including Damascus, Tartous, and Latakia—as well as areas retaken by the state, including Homs, parts of Aleppo, Dera'a, and Eastern Ghouta—there is rising unemployment, and poverty rates exceed 80 percent, with bread and fuel queues increasingly common (Osman 2020).

The health system is heavily centralized, with a greater number of services and investment in the major cities including Damascus, Aleppo, Latakia, and Homs (Abbara et al. 2015). The public sector in these areas remains the main health system, though the private sector is increasingly prominent. Figure 2.2 shows an organizational chart of the Ministry of Health, which sits in Damascus. The setup illustrates that decision-making power is mostly concentrated around four main positions: the health minister, the deputy minister for technical and medical affairs, the deputy minister for pharmaceutical and drug affairs, and the deputy minister for administrative and financial affairs.[1] The Ministry of Health consists of twenty-nine directorates of health across Syria, with no directorate for older people or for women. There is limited intersectoral or interdisciplinary collaboration within and across directorates.

Poor coordination, poor planning, and inequitable distribution of resources for health can be explained by weak governance mechanisms, corruption, and poor strategic planning from the Ministry of Health. Alongside inadequate coordination within the health sector is insufficient intersectoral coordination between ministries or directorates relevant to health, including education, social affairs, agriculture, and water. Figure 2.3 shows the flow of funds and responsibilities among ministries. There is a lack of transparency in how health or humanitarian aid is distributed

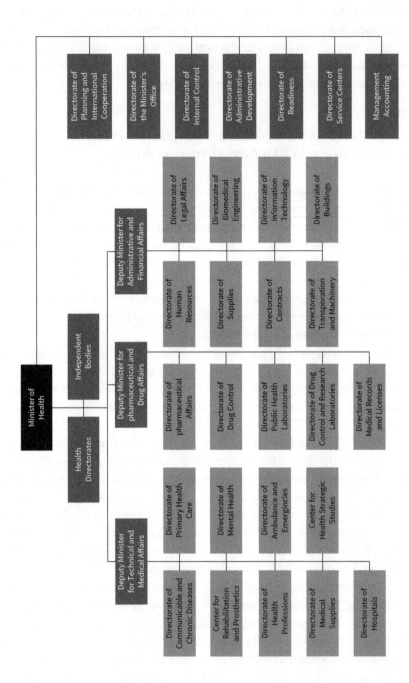

Figure 2.2. This figure shows the structure of the Ministry of Health and relevant directorates, translated from Arabic.

Source: "وزارة الصحة." 2019. Moh.Gov.Sy. http://www.moh.gov.sy/Default.aspx?tabid=102&language=ar-YE.

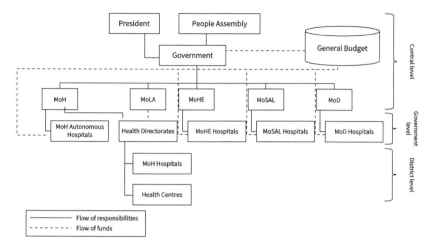

Figure 2.3. This figure shows the flow of funds and responsibilities among various ministries and health centers at the central, governorate, and district levels. MoH— Ministry of Health. MoLA—Ministry of Local Administration. MoHE—Ministry of Higher Education. MoSAL—Ministry of Social Affairs and Labor. MoD—Ministry of Defense. *Source:* Kasturi, Sen. 2012. "Syria—Neoliberal Reforms in Health Sector Financing: Embedding Unequal Access?" *Social Medicine* 6 (3). https://www.researchgate.net/publication/277808894_Syria_Neoliberal_ Reforms_in_Health_Sector_Financing_Embedding_Unequal_Access.

to some populations; for example, there have been accusations that those who are known to be against the Syrian government or who were previously under opposition control have received poor services or provisions for health (Chatham House 2019). For women and other vulnerable groups, there is an absence of intersectional gender considerations in the aims or objectives of the Ministry of Health, affecting both the employment of women in health as well as women as healthcare seekers (Kherallah et al. 2012).[2]

HEALTH CARE ACCESS THROUGH THE PUBLIC AND PRIVATE SECTORS

The public healthcare sector in areas under Syrian government control is within the scope of the Ministry of Health and public university hospitals such as Al Mwasat, and Assad University Hospital in Damascus. The ministry has the role of coordinating and managing public health services. Other ministries also are involved in decision-making, such as the Ministry of Social Affairs and Labor, the Ministry of Higher Education, the

Ministry of Defense, and the Ministry of Local Administration (Kherallah et al. 2012).

The private sector accounts for an estimated 40 percent of healthcare services through private hospitals, clinics, and pharmacies (Taleb et al. 2014). These are concentrated in the main cities of Damascus, Aleppo, Homs, Tartous, and Latakia. Poor regulation of the private sector has resulted in variable quality, high costs, and poor geographical spread, with concentration in urban rather than rural areas, and with poor correlation to the needs of the population. However, the weakened state of the public sector drives patients to seek private care if they can afford it, often at the expense of other essentials. Some healthcare workers are part of both the public and private sectors, which also may contribute to poor quality in the public sector as regulation to ensure attendance may be weak. Figure 2.4 shows 2019 Ministry of Health data for the number of hospitals per fifty thousand people for twelve of fourteen governorates across Syria; Idlib and Raqqa have not been included ("Health Statistical Abstract" 2019). The ministry estimates the number of doctors and nurses who provide care in the private sector, and the number of private versus public facilities, though data may be inaccurate and out of date given rapidly changing situations on the ground. This is particularly pertinent given reports of deaths of healthcare workers from COVID-19 during the 2020 pandemic (Human Rights Watch 2020b).

Though public health facilities were the main healthcare providers both before and after the onset of conflict, the health care provided was poor (Kherallah et al. 2012). These facilities include primary healthcare centers known as "Mostawsaf" or "Markaz Sehi," public hospitals, hospitals affiliated with universities, and military hospitals. The geographic distribution

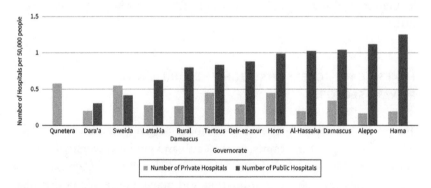

Figure 2.4. The number of hospitals per 50,000 people in the public and private sectors across governorates in areas under the control of the government of Syria (Ministry of Health data; 2019). Note that this is the number of hospitals rather than hospital beds.
Source: "Health Statistical Abstract 15th Issue." 2019. Moh.Gov.Sy. http://www.moh.gov.sy/LinkClick. aspx?fileticket=DqG7Iy5-sG8%3d&portalid=0&language=ar-YE.

favored urban versus rural areas, and hospital-based rather than community services. Patients avoided them if they could afford other care due to the low quality of care, long waiting times, and insufficient supply of medications and medical equipment (WHO 2006; Mershed et al. 2012). This was particularly the case in secondary and tertiary care, where waiting times were long unless patients had "Wasta," or connections, to move ahead in the queue. Due to the centralization of centers in larger urban settings, barriers to accessing cancer care included distance and the cost of transport.

THE ROLE OF INTERNATIONAL AND NONGOVERNMENTAL ORGANIZATIONS

The influence of international organizations operating through Damascus (including the World Health Organization, UNICEF, the UN High Commissioner for Refugees, the UN Relief and Works Agency, the UN Development Program, the International Committee of the Red Cross, and the International Federation of Red Cross and Red Crescent Societies) and a limited number of NGOs has increased during the conflict, and most are mandated to work with the Syrian government. As a result, there have been allegations of undue government influence on the work of these organizations and a lack of equity in the distribution of health or humanitarian aid and resources (Chatham House 2019). This has affected funding, with some international donors lecting to avoid donating directly to the Syrian government, preferring instead to go through NGOs registered in Damascus as intermediaries.

Accusations of corruption and preferential treatment for certain NGOs is prevalent. Before the conflict there were restrictions on civil society (Alzoubi 2017), and the only NGO allowed to operate without suppression or restriction was the Syria Trust for Development, established in 2006 by the Syrian president's wife, Asma Al Assad (Sinjab 2010). In 2016, it was revealed that the UN High Commissioner for Refugees had supported the trust with several million US dollars (Chatham House 2019). Other than the Syria Trust for Development, the other major NGO operating in areas controlled by the Syrian government is the Syrian Arab Red Crescent (SARC), which has close ties to the Syrian government, and through which around 60 percent of international aid reaching Syria is channeled (Syria Justice and Accountability Centre 2019). Since the start of the conflict, only a handful of other NGOs, also closely connected to the Syrian government, have received authorization from the Ministry of Foreign Affairs to work under the supervision of SARC, potentially so the government can maintain influence over their work. International or local NGOs that have tried to distribute health and humanitarian aid equitably in government-controlled areas during the conflict—including Médecins Sans Frontières (MSF), Save the Children, and Mercy Corps—have been evicted from these areas (Sparrow 2018). Concerns have been raised that areas retaken by the Syrian government have restricted access to health care, compared with areas that have remained loyal to the state. This interference as well as the potential effects of sanctions requires further study to verify, though political and security concerns may prevent this.

Chronic Neglect: The Health System in Northeast Syria

Northeast Syria encompasses an area of about 50,000 square kilometers and consists of the following self-governing subregions: Jazira, Euphrates, Raqqa, Tabqa, Manbij, and Deir Ezzor. According to the Syrian government's administrative division, it lies on parts of the Al-Hasakah, Raqqa, Deir Ezzor, and Aleppo governorates (Allsop and van Wilgenburg 2019). It is east of the Euphrates, bordering Turkey in the north, and Iraq and Kurdistan Iraq in the southeast. The health system in this area was underdeveloped and under-resourced even before the conflict; this has affected its ability to meet the needs of the population postconflict and, now, after the closure of the Yarubieh border crossing, during the COVID-19 pandemic (Human Rights Watch 2020a).

This region's ethnic makeup has transitioned over time and differs from that in other parts of Syria; the main ethnic groups currently are Kurds, Arabs, and Assyrians, with smaller populations of Armenians, Turkmen, and Circassians. Further demographic changes have occurred with the entry of hundreds of thousands of internally displaced people (IDPs) from other parts of Syria and from Iraq, after the Islamic State of Iraq and Levant's (ISIL) invasion of the latter (Allsop and van Wilgenburg 2019). Since 2012, northeast Syria has been under the control of the Kurdish-led Autonomous Administration of North and East Syria (AANES) and its armed wing, the Syrian Democratic Forces (SDF). In 2014, the United States allied with the People's Protection Unit (YPG), a Kurdish armed group (though some foreign fighters and Arabs have joined) against ISIL. This area remains volatile, with a number of groups with competing interests—including the United States, Russia, Turkey, and the Kurds—represented.

In 2019, northeast Syria had an estimated three million people (OCHA 2019a); of these, more than half, around 1.8 million, are in need of health and humanitarian aid (OCHA 2019a). The area hosts almost 710,000 internally displaced people, of whom around 91,000 live in camps in sub-optimal conditions, with limited services and liberties. Al Hol camp, which lies close to the Syria–Iraq border (and where the wives and children of ISIL members reside), is the largest in northeast Syria, with an estimated 65,000 IDPs living in it (Saad 2020); other camps are Areesha, Mahmoudli, Newroz, and Roj. After the withdrawal of US troops from the area, Turkey invaded, forcing 200,000 more people from their homes; of these, 129,000 have been able to return to their homes, but 70,590 individuals from Al-Hasakah, Ar-Raqqa, and Aleppo governorates could not return and remain internally displaced (OCHA 2019c). Three new informal IDP camps were established in northeast Syria as a response to the most recent displacements: Tweineh (hosting an estimated 4,120 people), Tal-Samen (hosting an estimated twenty people), and Daham (hosting an estimated 1,800 people).[49] Security concerns have forced the closure of the main local hospitals in Ras Al-Ain and Tal Abyad, and of two health centers in Tal Abyad, after the Turkish operation in October 2019 (WHO 2020b; OCHA 2019b).

UNDERDEVELOPED HEALTH SYSTEM IN NORTHEAST SYRIA

Those who support the Autonomous Administration of North and East Syria (AAES) describe it as having a democratic, decentralized government based on libertarian socialist ideologies embracing gender equality and pluralistic tolerance for other religions. In practice, however, it has been accused of authoritarianism and war crimes given its treatment of non-Kurdish populations in the area (Azeez 2019). The health system is organized by the Health and Environment Authority centrally and through subregional health committees; as such, it is one of few examples of a decentralized subnational health system in Syria. Professional organizations have emerged in northeast Syria; for example, Al-Jazeera Region Doctors' Union is equivalent to the Syrian Syndicate of medical doctors in government-controlled areas. These unions provide contracts with registered doctors to treat people working for the SDF in a health insurance–like scheme.

Even before the conflict, areas in Syria's northeast suffered from poor investment in the health system, and it remains under-resourced and underdeveloped compared with those in other regions. There is one public hospital in each of the major cities, with primary-care centers available in the smaller cities; however, the health system suffers from limited resources and insufficient staffing across all facilities. As in other parts of Syria, there are increasing numbers of private clinics. There is little regulation or oversight, however, resulting in variable quality across facilities.

Shortages of medical supplies and healthcare workers are widespread despite the high needs of the area's population. As in other parts of Syria, medical needs include communicable and noncommunicable disease care; maternal, neonatal, and child health services; and particularly, mental health and psychosocial support, given the degree of violence seen in this area. Violence has been perpetrated by all parties, including sexual and gender-based violence, leading to high levels of trauma among the population; this includes among children born into ISIL families who may have witnessed extreme violence or been forced to fight (Yayan 2019). Shortages of essential medicines in this area, as well as suspicion about the quality of generic or free medication, can lead those who have the means to pay out of pocket for services or medicines (UK Department for International Development 2018). A survey conducted in December 2017 in six governorates across Syria, including some in the northeast, found that almost two thirds of the population needed to pay out of pocket to access health care through the private sector, and in some areas almost 90 percent of the population were forced to pay out of pocket (UK Department for International Development 2018). International and local NGOs such as the Kurdish Red Crescent increasingly support medical services. But the intensification of violence, including attacks on health facilities, has forced some international organizations, including some MSF teams, to pull out (MSF 2019).

Health care is also adversely affected by damage to infrastructure, particularly water infrastructure, contributing to poor water, sanitation, and hygiene (WASH) and increases in communicable diseases. This presents particular challenges during the COVID-19 pandemic. In October 2019, Turkey and Turkish-backed forces took control of the Allouk water station, located near Ras Al-Ain (Human Rights Watch 2020c). This station provides water for 460,000 people in Al-Hasakah, including those already vulnerable in the Al Hol and Areesheh camps (Human Rights Watch 2020c). Hand washing is one of the few low-cost, feasible interventions for COVID-19 prevention in Syria and is already embedded within Syrian culture, with ablutions part of the pre-prayer ritual for Muslims; as such, this is a habit more people would adhere to if WASH is guaranteed. It would also have positive secondary benefits, including a reduction in other communicable diseases and childhood morbidity and mortality.

Splintered and Underfunded: The Health System in Northwest Syria

Northwest Syria is home to some of the last areas that remain outside Syrian government control. As of August 2020, this area contained an estimated 4.1 million people, of whom 2.7 million were IDPs; more than 76 percent of the population were women and children (UNHCR 2020; "Syrian Arab Republic: Recent Developments" 2020). Between December 2019 and February 2020, almost one million civilians were internally displaced after an escalation of hostilities (Syria Public Health Network 2020). Military operations continue in the area, with ongoing shelling, particularly around the M4 highway; this has resulted in hazardous explosives being a risk to civilians.

Travel in and out of this area is severely restricted. Cross-border travel to Turkey is increasingly difficult, not only due to restrictions related to the COVID-19 pandemic but also to the increasing control of border crossings. Cross-line movement between areas in northwest Syria under opposition control and areas under government control is limited, though the border between northwest Syria and areas in the north under Turkish control have more mobility across them. At present, the only border crossing for health and humanitarian provisions is through Bab Al-Hawa, which allows supplies from Turkey to the northwest; but there is no guarantee that the UN Security Council will renew its cross-border resolution in July 2021, given the increasing threat of a veto from China and Russia. If this border crossing is not renewed, humanitarian aid for over 2.8 million people will be severely hindered (OCHA 2020a), with concerns that aid supplied through Damascus will not flow to these areas.

The evolution of the health system in northwest Syria differs from that in other areas due to its geographic location, which leaves it sandwiched between Turkey and areas controlled by the Syrian government; its acceptance of large numbers of IDPs who have fled from other areas; and the role of external funders and humanitarian organizations. Soon after the escalation of violence and the entry of IDPs from other parts of Syria, NGOs began to form both within the area and in Turkey. Because of the slow response from the international community, local Syrian and expatriate Syrian NGOs were among the first responders; these included organizations such as the Syrian American Medical Society, the Syrian Expatriate Medical Association, the Union of Medical Care and Relief Organizations (UOSSM), Syria Relief and Development, and Hand in Hand for Aid and Development, with international NGOs and organizations later joining and basing themselves in Gaziantep, in Turkey (OCHA 2020b). To improve response coordination and strengthen the voice of Syrian NGOs, some NGOs formed a coalition called the Syrian NGO Alliance ("Syrian NGO Alliance" 2020). As international NGOs started to arrive, they partnered with Syrian organizations that had more established and trusted links within Syria, and through which they could work (Duclos et al. 2019). Due to their established records, these international NGOs could attract funding early in the response that some Syrian NGOs could not. The cross-border delivery of humanitarian aid was initially more straightforward, with more porous borders between Turkey and Syria. These borders have become increasingly policed, though the smuggling of people and goods continues.

The WHO-led Health Cluster, based in Gaziantep, includes international NGOs and Syrian NGOs and holds powers around decision-making for healthcare services in northwest Syria. Its aim is to provide leadership, coordination, and accountability for health and other relevant sectors, including protection, nutrition, and logistics. Yet, particularly early in the humanitarian response, unilateral, often funder-driven, decision-making by NGOs resulted in poor distribution of services; this, in turn, led to gaps and overlaps in healthcare provision (OCHA 2018). Power imbalances and different strategies among stakeholders—including the Health Cluster, health directorates, local councils, quasi-governmental bodies, and healthcare providers based in the northwest—have led to increasing fragmentation across the sector. Local actors also have faced challenges with regard to funding (particularly long-term or sustainable funding) and legitimacy in the eyes of donors, mostly due to their lack of an established track record, financial records, or governance structures that would make them eligible for certain funding streams. This has resulted in a variety of models through which health facilities have been established, funded, and managed.

The subnational health system in this area, as in other areas of Syria, has suffered from weak leadership; this includes the Syrian Interim Government (SIG), which established a Ministry of Health and adopted health directorates under its remit. The SIG became less prominent as NGOs gained funding and prominence. Other actors in the northwest, such as the Salvation Government (a group with links to the group Hayat Tahrir Alsham), have also established a Ministry of Health, though it has had limited influence on the ground, leading to an increasingly politicized climate for health. Locally, health directorates have been established, but these have functioned with mixed success, with disagreements and competition among key actors. For example, in the Aleppo governorate, clashes and competition between the Aleppo City Medical Council (mostly focused on Aleppo city) and the Free Medical Union (mostly focused on rural areas) affected the ability to establish an effective Health Directorate there (Physicians for Human Rights 2015). Though neither the Aleppo City Medical Council nor the Free Medical Union survived, challenges remain within the Aleppo Health Directorate.

The health of the population in this area is heavily affected by attacks on healthcare facilities, inadequate WASH, and insufficient specialized services—for example, maternal and child health, oncology, and dialysis—to meet the population's needs. This has been exacerbated by the COVID-19 pandemic, because funding and resources have been diverted to this emergency response, affecting the availability of funds and human resources for other medical services. There are simply not enough healthcare workers, particularly specialists; figures from the Idlib Health Directorate estimate that there are around one thousand doctors and two thousand nurses and midwives in the entire northwest Syria region. This equates to eight healthcare staff per ten thousand people, which is below the minimum recommendation set by the Sphere humanitarian standards community of twenty-two healthcare staff per ten thousand people (WHO 2020a). Though initiatives in this area aim to support healthcare-worker education, there exist concerns about quality, sustainability, and the recognition of qualifications obtained in certain academic institutions (Bdaiwi et al. 2020). There is also concern about the number of informally trained healthcare workers, who were essential at the start of the conflict, but who, as the conflict has become increasingly protracted, have found themselves without qualifications or opportunities for work, particularly as the humanitarian response has become professionalized.

Underexplored: The Health System in Areas Under Turkish Control

There is very little publicly available information about the health system in areas occupied by Turkish Armed Forces and the Syrian National Army since 2016, so we draw heavily on information from key informants. This area includes locations formerly under the control of ISIL, including Afrin, Al-Bab, Azaz, Tal Abyad, and Ras al-Ayn. The health system in this area is primarily governed by Turkish directorates along the northern border of Syria. Although Syrian health directorates still exist in the main towns, their role has been diminished and disempowered by the Turkish authorities. Over the last four years, the Turkish health directorates have contributed to the establishment of new hospitals and health centers in line with Turkish standards elsewhere in Turkey, including four health centers in the northern Aleppo governorate.[3] All hospitals and health facilities are managed by Turkish nationals, while health staff (medical doctors and nurses) are predominantly Syrian. The quality of care is reported to be good within

Table 2.1 FUNDERS AND OVERSEERS OF AREAS WITHIN TURKISH CONTROL

Town	Governed by	Health Services Financed by
Azaz and Al Raai	Kilis Health Directorate	Turkish Ministry of Health
Al- Bab and Jarabulus	Gaziantep Health Directorate	(Ankara)
Tell Abyad and Ras-al-Ayn	Urfa Health Directorate	

these services and is provided without discrimination to both Arab and Kurdish populations. The Turkish government has allowed some NGOs (Syria Relief and Development, UOSSM, and the Independent Doctors' Association) to establish primary-care and maternity centers in these areas, to support the provision of care to the population (see Table 2.1).

An important emerging challenge in this area is the poor coordination between health authorities in the Turkish-controlled areas and health authorities in northwest Syria, whose populations share a border. This is particularly crucial when it comes to health surveillance and communication regarding communicable diseases of public health importance, such as COVID-19, where porous borders could increase spread between the two areas. For example, COVID-19 cases were identified in the Al-Bab district in the Aleppo governorate, which is under Turkish control; but there was no collaboration or cooperation with the Early Warning and Response Network surveillance system team, which is active in northwest Syria in non-Turkish-controlled areas. Other challenges include bureaucracy due to the nature of the Turkish health system, where most decisions require approval by the Ankara Ministry of Health, which can cause significant delays. Further evaluation of the health system in this area, and of its responsiveness to and interaction with other areas, particularly northwest Syria, is needed.

THE COVID-19 PANDEMIC AS A STRESSOR ON SYRIA'S SUBNATIONAL HEALTH SYSTEMS

The COVID-19 pandemic has further exposed and exacerbated fractures within and between the various subnational health systems across Syria. Populations faced with protracted conflict and crises as in Syria have faced numerous challenges in responding to COVID-19, with destroyed infrastructure and healthcare facilities, inadequate shelter and WASH, and insufficient quality and quantity of healthcare workers impeding the public health response. Cases of COVID-19 in countries neighboring Syria, including Lebanon, were announced as early as February 2020. Syria closed its borders on March 23, a delay that could have led to the entry of cases, particularly from Iran, with which Syria had close political ties up to that point (Abbara et al. 2020).

The first case of COVID-19 in Syria was confirmed on March 22, in Damascus, with cases declared in northeast Syria in April 2020 and in northwest Syria in July 2020. The response in each area has differed, though there have been common challenges: the politicization of the response, insufficient testing capacity, insufficient resources including personal protective equipment (PPE), insufficient numbers of COVID-19 isolation or inpatient beds, and poor compliance with public health measures such as face coverings, quarantine, self-isolation, and hand washing (Abbara et al. 2020). Though there have been good examples of community-led initiatives (Ekzayez 2020), there has been some resistance from a population that continues to face ongoing violence. Lockdown measures and school closures were poorly enforced across the country, with concerns that they exacerbated mental health and psychosocial challenges, financial strains in a population and economy reliant on informal labor, poverty, and protection measures.

In areas under Syrian government control, the health system is ill-equipped to respond to COVID-19, and evidence suggests that the extent of the outbreak has been suppressed for political reasons. For example, as of the end of November 2020, Syria had declared around 7,000 cases, compared with 120,000 in Lebanon, 198,000 in Jordan, 468,000 in Turkey, and 908,000 in Iran. The WHO has supported healthcare workers' training and the delivery of PPE and polymerase chain reaction (PCR) testing supplies to Damascus, with the intention that these be distributed to areas under Syrian government control and, after the closure of the Yarubieh border crossing, to northeast Syria. Most of the resources, however, have been used to support areas under Syrian government control, affecting the COVID-19 response in the northeast, an area that already has faced chronic underinvestment in the health system.

In northwest Syria, the fragmented health system and the slow response despite the early establishment of a WHO-led COVID-19 Task Force there—alongside insufficient testing capacity, resources, and healthcare workers, as well as weak leadership and governance—has adversely affected this area's ability to stem the virus's spread. Despite an initially slow rise, the number of cases in the northwest has increased rapidly, and the health system is overwhelmed; this could lead to indirect deaths from other conditions, or from insufficient availability of inpatient care or resources for COVID-19 patients.

Healthcare Workers in Syria: Casualties of Politics and Pandemics

Even before the COVID-19 pandemic, Syria's healthcare workers faced numerous challenges during the course of the conflict. The deliberate targeting of healthcare workers has been a hallmark of the conflict since the peaceful uprisings began, and thousands have either had their training interrupted, have been forcibly displaced (either internally or as refugees), or have been killed or imprisoned in the course of their work (Bdaiwi et al. 2020). More than 923 healthcare workers have been killed directly during the conflict, with more than 90 percent killed by the Syrian government and its allies (Physicians for Human Rights 2020).

These factors have contributed to the forced exodus of healthcare workers, leaving those who remain in Syria working in even more challenging conditions, where understaffing is common and there are gaps in specialist training. In areas outside government control, the lack of recognition or accreditation of healthcare worker training, including at the university level, presents a challenge for the quality of training and for healthcare workers who wish to remain in Syria (Bdaiwi et al. 2020). During the COVID-19 pandemic, there have been frequent reports of deaths of healthcare workers, which are suspected to be due to COVID-19, though these have not been formally confirmed, particularly in government-controlled areas. On August 16, 2020, a list of sixty-one healthcare workers who died from COVID-19 in government-controlled areas of Syria was released on Facebook, the real number is probably much higher.[4]

Concerns regarding the availability, training, and geographic distribution of healthcare workers across Syria existed before the conflict, but all these matters have been adversely affected by the impact of the conflict on the health system. For example, preconflict, there was a greater concentration of doctors in urban rather than rural areas, with a greater number of physicians in some regions compared with others. In the Tartous and Latakia governorates, for instance, the number of physicians per one thousand people was seven times higher than in Dera'a or rural Damascus ("Health Statistical Abstract" 2019). The conflict has exacerbated such differences, with significantly fewer healthcare workers of the right quality, quantity, and specialization essential both now and in the postconflict period. Given the time and resources it takes to train physician and nonphysician healthcare workers and the changing needs of a population in a fragmented and under-resourced health system under, urgent investment is required at all levels of health-worker training to properly meet the needs of the future health system.

From fragmentation to collaboration

The protracted conflict in Syria has fragmented the country's health system, resulting in at least four subnational health systems within its borders. There is little communication or collaboration between these health systems, which limits opportunities for cross-learning or responding to the needs of the population. The COVID-19 pandemic has shown how important such communication is. As we begin to think about the post-conflict period, research analyzing and comparing differences between the health systems is needed, as are mechanisms for increased collaboration. In addition, research exploring context-driven interventions is essential to inform policies around Syria's future health system.

As we look to the future, it is likely that at least low-level violence will continue. It is also likely that fragmentation of the health system will remain, at least to some extent. Health initiatives that can be delivered in different areas in Syria—for example, relating to maternal health or midwifery training—with some local adaptation could be one way to address some of this fragmentation. Importantly, it is not only the health system that is fragmented, but society as well, given the detrimental effects of the conflict on communities and social structures. As such, community-led approaches are essential for empowering communities during recovery and establishing responsive health systems. Given the high health burdens among populations across Syria, inclusive approaches such as universal healthcare coverage (in line with the United Nations' Sustainable Development Goals) will be essential to the population's recovery. All of this requires political will, and clear leadership and governance across the health and other related sectors. Without such measures, the health system will remain fragmented and unable to respond effectively to the Syrian population's needs.

ACKNOWLEDGMENTS

We would like to thank the following for their contributions to the conceptualization of this chapter and for providing information: Dr. Abdulkareem Ekzayez, Dr. Ola Faham, Dr. Omar Al Hiraki, Dr. Naser Mhawesh, Dr. Mahmoud Hariri, Dr. Enrico Pavignani, and Dr. Samer Jabbour.

NOTES

1. "الهيكل التنظيمي." 2019. Moh.Gov.Sy. http://www.moh.gov.sy/Default. aspx?tabid=105&language=ar-YE.
2. "مهام الوزارة." 2019. Moh.Gov.Sy. http://www.moh.gov.sy/Default. aspx?tabid=102&language=ar-YE.
3. "افتتاح مركز صحي في بلدة الراعي بحلب." 2017. SMART News Agency. https://bit.ly/ 2Jl7CgW.
4. "قائمة باسماء 61 من خيرة الأطباء الذين خسرتهم سورية في الآيام الماضية." 2020. Facebook.Com. https://www.facebook.com/halab2019/posts/ 1323427528001319?_rdc=1&_rdr.

REFERENCES

Abbara, Aula, Karl Blanchet, Zaher Sahloul, Fouad, Adam Coutts, and Wasim Maziak. 2015. "The Effect of the Conflict on Syria's Health System and Human Resources for Health." *World Health & Population 16* (1). https://beta. longwoods.com/content/24318.

Abbara, Aula, Diana Rayes, Ola Fahham, Omar Alrashid Alhiraki, Munzer Khalil, Abdulrahman Alomar, and Ahmad Tarakji. 2020. "Coronavirus 2019 and Health Systems Affected by Protracted Conflict: The Case of Syria." *International Journal of Infectious Diseases 96*: 192–95.

Allsopp, Harriet, and Wladimir van Wilgenburg. 2019. *The Kurds of Northern Syria: Governance, Diversity and Conflicts.* London: I. B. Tauris.

Alzoubi, Zedoun. 2017. "Syrian Civil Society during the Peace Talks in Geneva: Role and Challenges." *New England Journal of Public Policy 29* (1). https:// scholarworks.umb.edu/cgi/viewcontent.cgi?referer=https://scholar.google. com/&httpsredir=1&article=1710&context=nejpp.

Azeez, Govand Khalid. 2019. "The 'Kurd' between Capitalist-Statist Nationalism and Class Conflict." *Critique (Glasgow) 47* (3): 411–32.

Yamama Bdaiwi, Diana Rayes, Ammar Sabouni, Lina Murad, Fouad, Waseem Zakaria, Mahmoud Hariri, Abdelkarim Ekzayez, Ahmad Tarakji, and Aula Abbara. 2020. "Challenges of Providing Healthcare Worker Education and Training in Protracted Conflict: A Focus on Non–government Controlled Areas in North West Syria." *Conflict and Health 14*: 1505–1752.

Chatham House. 2019. "Principled Aid in Syria: A Framework for International Agencies." https://www.chathamhouse.org/sites/default/files/2019-07-04- PrincipledAidSyria.pdf.

Duclos, Diane, Abdulkarim Ekzayez, Fatima Ghaddar, Francesco Checchi, and Karl Blanchet. 2019. "Localisation and Cross-Border Assistance to Deliver Humanitarian Health Services in North-West Syria: A Qualitative Inquiry for The Lancet-AUB Commission on Syria." *Conflict and Health 13* (1): 20.

Ekzayez, Abdulkarim, Munzer al-Khalil, Mohamad Jasiem, Raed Al Saleh, Zedoun Alzoubi, Kristen Meagher, and Preeti Patel. 2020. "COVID-19 response in northwest Syria: Innovation and community engagement in a complex conflict." *Journal of Public Health, 42*(3), 504–509.

Fouad M. Fouad, Annie Sparrow, Ahmad Tarakji, Mohamad Alameddine, Prof Fadi El-Jardali, Adam P Coutts, Nour El Arnaout, Lama Bou Karroum, Mohammed

Jawad, Sophie Roborgh, Aula Abbara, Fadi Alhalabi, and Ibrahim AlMasri. 2017. "Health Workers and the Weaponisation of Health Care in Syria: A Preliminary Inquiry for The Lancet–American University of Beirut Commission on Syria." *The Lancet 390* (10111): 2516–526.

Guha-Sapir, Debarati, Benjamin Schlüter, Jose Manuel Rodriguez-Llanes, Louis Lillywhite, and Madelyn Hsiao-Rei Hicks. 2018. "Patterns of Civilian and Child Deaths Due to War-Related Violence in Syria: A Comparative Analysis from the Violation Documentation Center Dataset, 2011–16." *The Lancet Global Health 6* (1): E103–E110.

"Health Statistical Abstract 15th Issue." 2019. *Moh.Gov.Sy.* http://www.moh.gov.sy/ LinkClick.aspx?fileticket=DqG7Iy5-sG8%3d&portalid=0&language=ar-YE.

Human Rights Watch. 2020a. "Syria: Aid Restrictions Hinder Covid-19 Response." https://www.hrw.org/news/2020/04/28/ syria-aid-restrictions-hinder-covid-19-response.

Human Rights Watch. 2020b. "Syria: Health Workers Lack Protection in Pandemic." https://www.hrw.org/news/2020/09/02/ syria-health-workers-lack-protection-pandemic.

Human Rights Watch. 2020c. "Turkey/Syria: Weaponizing Water in Global Pandemic?" https://www.hrw.org/news/2020/03/31/turkey/ syria-weaponizing-water-global-pandemic.

Kherallah, Mazen, Tayeb Alahfez, Zaher Sahloul, Khaldoun Dia Eddin, and Ghyath Jamil. 2012. "Health Care in Syria before and during the Crisis." *Avicenna Journal of Medicine 2* (3): 51–53.

Mershed, Mania, Reinhard Busse, and Ewout Ginneken. 2012. "Healthcare Financing in Syria: Satisfaction with the Current System and the Role of National Health Insurance—a Qualitative Study of Householders' Views." *International Journal of Health Planning and Management 27* (2): 167–79.

Mowafi, Hani, and Jennifer Leaning. 2018. "Documenting Deaths in the Syrian War." *The Lancet Global Health 6* (1): E14–E15.

MSF (Médecins Sans Frontières). 2019. "Northeast Syria: MSF forced to evacuate staff due to extreme volatility in the region." Press release. https://www.msf. org/northeast-syria-msf-forced-evacuate-staff-due-extreme-volatility-region.

OCHA. 2018. "Major UN Aid Deliver to Syria from Jordan." Press release. https:// www.humanitarianresponse.info/sites/www.humanitarianresponse.info/files/ documents/files/ocha_jordan_press_release.pdf.

OCHA. 2019a. "Northeast Syria—As Half a Million People Gradually Regain Access to Safe Water—The Number of Displaced People Nears 180,000 [EN/AR]." https://reliefweb.int/report/syrian-arab-republic/ northeast-syria-half-million-people-gradually-regain-access-safe-water.

OCHA. 2019b. "Syria—Flash Update #5, Humanitarian Impact of the Military Operation in North-Eastern Syria, 14 October 2019 [EN/AR]." *OCHA* situation report. https://reliefweb.int/report/syrian-arab-republic/ syria-flash-update-5-humanitarian-impact-military-operation-north.

OCHA. 2019c. "Syrian Arab Republic: North East Syria Displacement." https://reliefweb.int/map/syrian-arab-republic/ syrian-arab-republic-north-east-syria-displacement-18-december-2019.

OCHA. 2020a. "Recent Developments in Northwest Syria— Situation Report No. 20—as of 9 September 2020." Situation report. https://reliefweb.int/report/syrian-arab-republic/ recent-developments-northwest-syria-situation-report-no-20-9-september.

OCHA. 2020b. "Annual Report—2019 Humanitarian Response Plan for Syria—28 October 2020." https://www.humanitarianresponse.info/operations/whole-of-syria.

OCHA. 2020c. "Syrian Arab Republic: United Nations Cross-Border Operations under UNSC Resolutions." https://reliefweb.int/sites/reliefweb.int/files/resources/cnv_syr_xb_regional_jun2020_200708_en.pdf.

Omar, Abdulaziz. 2020. "Understanding and Preventing Attacks on Health Facilities During Armed Conflict in Syria." *Risk Management and Healthcare Policy* 13: 191–203.

Osman, Nadda. 2020. "Syrians Forced into Cages to Queue for Bread." *Middle East Eye*. https://www.middleeasteye.net/news/syria-cages-queue-bread-condemnation.

Physicians for Human Rights. 2015. "Aleppo Abandoned" A Case Study on Health Care in Syria." https://reliefweb.int/sites/reliefweb.int/files/resources/aleppo-abandoned.pdf.

Physicians for Human Rights. 2020. "Medical Personnel Are Targeted in Syria." https://phr.org/our-work/resources/medical-personnel-are-targeted-in-syria/.

Saad, Neil J. 2020. "The Al Hol Camp in Northeast Syria: Health and Humanitarian Challenges." *BMJ Global Health* 5 (7): E002491.

St. Andrews, University of. 2017. "Syria at War: Five Years On." https://www.unescwa.org/sites/www.unescwa.org/files/publications/files/syria-war-five-years.pdf.

Sinjab, Lina. "Is Syria Ready to Engage with Ngos?" 2010. *BBC News*. http://news.bbc.co.uk/2/hi/middle_east/8477748.stm.

Sparrow, Annie. 2018. "How UN Humanitarian Aid Has Propped Up Assad." *Foreign Affairs*. https://www.foreignaffairs.com/articles/syria/2018-09-20/how-un-humanitarian-aid-has-propped-assad.

Specia, Megan. "How Syria's Death Toll Is Lost in the Fog of War." *New York Times*, April 13, 2018. https://www.nytimes.com/2018/04/13/world/middleeast/syria-death-toll.html.

Syria Justice & Accountability Centre. 2019. "Inside the Syrian Arab Red Crescent." https://syriaaccountability.org/updates/2019/08/08/inside-the-syrian-arab-red-crescent/.

Syria Public Health Network. 2020. "Policy Brief North West Syria: Humanitarian Catastrophe." http://syriahealthnetwork.org/attachments/article/37/PolicyBrief_NWSyria_28.2.20.pdf.

"Syrian Arab Republic: Recent Developments in Northwest Syria, Situation Report No. 19—as of 21 August 2020." 2020. https://www.humanitarianresponse.info/sites/www.humanitarianresponse.info/files/documents/files/nw_syria_sitrep19_21aug2020.pdf.

Syrian Arab Republic UN Country Team. 2020. "Framework for the Immediate Socio-Economic Response to Covid-19." https://reliefweb.int/sites/reliefweb.int/files/resources/SYR_Socioeconomic-Response-Plan_2020B-compressed.pdf.

Syrian Observatory for Human Rights. 2020. "Syrian Revolution Nine Years On: 586,100 Persons Killed and Millions of Syrians Displaced and Injured." https://www.syriahr.com/en/157193/.

"Syrian NGO Alliance." 2020. *Reliefweb*. https://reliefweb.int/organization/syrian-ngo-alliance.

Taleb, Ziyad Ben, Raed Bahelah, Fouad M. Fouad, Adam Coutts, Meredith Wilcox, and Wasim Maziak. 2014. "Syria: Health in a Country Undergoing Tragic Transition." *International Journal of Public Health* 60 (S1): 63–72.

UK Department for International Development. 2018. "Protecting Healthcare in Syria." https://www.gov.uk/research-for-development-outputs/protecting-healthcare-in-syria.

UNHCR (United Nations High Commissioner for Refugees). 2020. "North-west Syria: Cross-Border Humanitarian Response Fact Sheet (July 2020)." Situation report. https://reliefweb.int/report/syrian-arab-republic/north-west-syria-cross-border-humanitarian-response-fact-sheet-july-2020.

WHO (World Health Organization). 2006. "Health System Profile—Syria." Regional Health Systems Observatory. http://digicollection.org/hss/documents/s17311e/s17311e.pdf.

WHO (World Health Organization). 2020a. "Health Resources Availability Monitoring System (Herams), Third Quarter, 2020 Report, Turkey Health Cluster for Syria, July-September 2020." Health Cluster. https://reliefweb.int/report/syrian-arab-republic/health-resources-availability-monitoring-system-herams-third-quarter-1.

WHO (World Health Organization). 2020b. "Health Sector Syria—Health Sector Bulletin—December 2019—Syrian Arab Republic." *Health Cluster,* situation report. https://reliefweb.int/report/syrian-arab-republic/health-sector-syria-health-sector-bulletin-december-2019.

WHO (World Health Organization). 2020c. "Polio Outbreak In Syria Successfully Stopped | Syria-News | Syrian Arab Republic." *Emro.Who.Int.* http://www.emro.who.int/syr/syria-news/polio-outbreak-successfully-stopped.html.

Yayan, Emriye Hilal, Mehmet Emin Düken, Aynur Aytekin Özdemir, and Ayda Çelebioğlu. 2019. "Mental Health Problems of Syrian Refugee Children: Post-Traumatic Stress, Depression and Anxiety." *Journal of Pediatric Nursing* 51: E27–E32.

CHAPTER 3

The Moral Norm, the Law, and the Limits of Protection for Wartime Medical Units

NEVE GORDON

In a 2019 fact sheet documenting the systematic attacks on medical infrastructure in Syria, the nongovernmental organization Physicians for Human Rights describes the Syrian government's eight-year attempt to "punish civilians residing in opposition-held territories, destroy their ability to survive, and draw them into government-held areas or drive them out of the country" (Physicians for Human Rights 2019). After offering a concise analysis of the assaults on health care, the rights group concludes that the attacks rise to the "level of war crimes" and "crimes against humanity." It then provides a series of recommendations, calling on all parties involved in the conflict to immediately end attacks on unlawful targets, including civilians, health facilities, and medical personnel; urging Russia, Turkey, and the United Nations to "maintain the de-militarized zone in northwest Syria"; and requesting that the United Nations and individual member states "maintain financial, political, and diplomatic support for efforts to document violations of international human rights and humanitarian law and principles, with insistence on justice and accountability for war crimes and crimes against humanity." Finally, the group calls on the "United Nations and states supporting a political solution to the Syrian conflict to integrate accountability into efforts to bring the conflict to an end, knowing that sustainable peace can only be built on the foundations of

Neve Gordon, *The Moral Norm, the Law, and the Limits of Protection for Wartime Medical Units* In: *Everybody's War*.
Edited by: Jehan Bseiso, Michiel Hofman, and Jonathan Whittall, Oxford University Press. © Médecins Sans Frontières
2021. DOI: 10.1093/oso/9780197514641.003.0004

justice" (Physicians for Human Rights 2019). In a similar vein, Safeguarding Health, a coalition of over forty national and international nongovernmental organizations, concludes in its report on Syria that "there is an urgent need for an effective cessation of hostilities and for accountability for these documented war crimes" (Safeguarding Health 2018).

Two themes stand out in reports published by humanitarian and human rights organizations such as those above: The main reference point for assessing, evaluating, and judging attacks on health care is international law, particularly international humanitarian law; and the primary way of redressing the law's violation and various forms of impunity is through legal accountability. Legal advocacy is, in other words, the principal strategy adopted by many human rights and humanitarian organizations in their struggle to protect health care in Syria. The same groups that are generally extremely critical about policies undermining human rights around the world appear, however, to refrain from serious self-reflection about the underlying assumptions of legal advocacy (Mutua 2001; Nagy 2008; Berkovitch and Gordon 2008), the benefits versus disadvantages of deploying international law as the key reference for evaluating actions (Drumbl 2007), the strategy's effectiveness (Kennedy 2005), the political structures it elides (Marks 2011), the power relations it reinforces (Douzinas 2007; Hopgood 2013), and alternative strategies that may be eclipsed in the process (Perugini and Gordon 2015). Legal advocacy has become a taken-for-granted strategy, a self-evident approach rather than one subjected to ongoing self-reflection and critical assessment.

Syria offers a case study by which to interrogate the relationship between international humanitarian law and the moral norm pertaining to health care in theaters of violence—namely, the idea that medical units should be protected during armed conflict. International humanitarian law emanates from a series of moral norms that together reflect a humanitarian ideal, and one of the law's roles is to reproduce and strengthen these norms (Meron 1989; Kennedy 2008). But does humanitarian law indeed help reinforce the moral norm offering medical units protection during war? Or, paradoxically, does the law play a role in undermining it? And if the law is detrimental to the norm, what might be the implications for legal advocacy?

To investigate the relation between the norm and the law, I briefly describe how the Syrian government transformed medical units into strategic targets. I then discuss the norm that informs the law and incites it to offer these units protections, showing that the norm itself frames health care as a neutral enterprise, distinct from and external to the war effort.[1] Next, I analyze the way the norm casts the relation between health care and war to underscore two related interpretive gaps. The first gap is the one between the way the norm frames the relation between health and war—namely, as distinct—and the way the actors in Syria understand this relation—namely, as inextricably linked. The second gap is inscribed in the legal provisions themselves. On the one hand, the law assumes the neutrality of health professionals; but at the same time it recognizes, through a list of exceptions, that health and war frequently overlap. The first gap, I argue, exposes the fragility of the norm dealing with medical units during war, while the second suggests that the norm's instability is not new, and that from the First Geneva Convention, in 1864, legal provisions dealing with medical units have helped undermine the very norm they were meant to sustain and reinforce. The question at stake is how all of the above might affect our approach to legal advocacy.

THE ASSAULT ON HEALTH CARE IN SYRIA

When Bashar al-Assad replaced his father to become Syria's president in July 2000, he promised to introduce a more open and progressive form of governance. Eleven years later, the image of civility Assad had been cultivating shattered as he sent security forces to crush popular protests in the southern part of the country (Munif 2020; Wedeen 2019; Pearlman 2017). As a plethora of humanitarian and human rights groups have documented, from the very beginning Assad's troops violated the legal articles that provide protections to medical units during conflict.[2]

The following description of the assault on health care in Syria is based on ninety-nine interviews with health workers—including doctors, paramedics, first aid providers, logisticians, and ambulance drivers—carried out by Médecins Sans Frontières (MSF) staff between July 2016 and March 2017. Interviewees included people from Syria's fourteen governorates, and the conversations covered events that took place between March 2011 and March 2017. For logistical, security, and strategic reasons, MSF staff had greater access to health workers from opposition-controlled areas, and thus their voices are afforded greater representation here. Some participants were inside Syria at the time of interview, so were contacted remotely, via Skype, WhatsApp, or phone, while others had left the country and were interviewed face-to-face in Turkey, Lebanon, Belgium, and the Netherlands. Eighty-seven interviews were conducted in Arabic, and the remaining twelve in English. For reasons of privacy and personal safety, the names of the interviewees and all information that might identify them have been redacted.[3]

The interviews highlight the precarity of the international norm establishing protections for medical units. Moreover, they suggest that the cartography of health care in Syria was transformed in three major phases, and that the government gradually securitized the provision of health and constituted the opposition's medical field as a threat that should be annihilated. In different regions within Syria these phases transpired during different periods, and often the phases—particularly the second and third—overlapped in time.

Phase 1: Health Providers as Active Agents in War

The first phase corresponded with the uprising's first months. In late March 2011, government soldiers began shooting at unarmed protesters in Daraa (Munif 2020). Injured people who reached the local hospital were arrested by security forces; some were taken to torture chambers, while others disappeared. Rapidly, an extremely disturbing process unfolded during which government health care institutions were transformed into traps used by security forces to capture protesters seeking aid.

The struggles during this phase were still not classified as armed conflict, and therefore international humanitarian provisions protecting the wounded and health staff did not apply. In addition, it is not uncommon for domestic laws to require hospitals to report the presence of patients with violent injuries to the police. Where the police serve the public interest, this can be acceptable. And the law usually prescribes that a patient cannot be arrested and transferred from a hospital without a doctor's consent. In this phase, though, the interviewees underscore that the government ignored the norm allowing patients uninterrupted treatment.

As the accounts of health professionals suggest, this propelled healthcare activists to develop creative solutions for delivering assistance, and they began establishing clandestine medical safe houses—in flats, basements, construction sites, and farms—to treat wounded protesters and sick people associated with the resistance in areas controlled by the government. Thus emerged an alternative first aid system operating alongside the government health system, within the same spatial terrain but hidden from government purview.

Describing the early days of the uprising, one aid worker from the Ghouta governorate explained how he and other health workers picked up protesters who'd been shot before government forces could get to them. "We built hidden health centers, and that was the biggest challenge at that time," he said. "We would take the patient to the health center, the doctor would treat him, and a nurse would follow up on his condition. Then we would move patients to another place in order to keep them safe as the regime was searching houses randomly. We would move patients during the night to safe places" (Interviewee 2001). A physician from Deir ez-Zor described a similar situation: "The regime had posted security men in each private or public hospital, a security 'filter' at the gate of each hospital which arrested any injured from the Free Syrian Army or the protesters. Any injured person whatsoever would be arrested, even before being treated, regardless of their condition." He proceeded to recount how a group of health professionals set up thirteen secret safe houses that served as makeshift medical centers. "The work," he explained, "was undertaken underground, in a strict secrecy which would shock you" (Interviewee 1017).

In the beginning, the medical safe houses were very basic, and there was little coordination among health professionals within each city. But as the government expanded its attacks against protesters, health professionals concerned about the welfare of the civilian population began coordinating and collaborating with one another. "I was surprised by the numbers of wounded people that I had to treat, which were less than the numbers of people wounded in the streets," said a neurosurgeon who lived in the Damascus governorate. "I figured out later on that other medical teams were also working in secret, but without any coordination with us or between each other. We sometimes also met those medical teams while treating the injured, and those meetings increased with the intensification of fighting, and then teams started collaborating" (Interviewee 1015).

During the first weeks of demonstrations, with injured protesters being arrested in hospitals, governmental medical institutions were rendered off limits to people resisting the government. But as the demonstrations continued, even staff members working in governmental hospitals suspected of secretly treating people aligned with the resistance were at risk. In a report published by an Independent International Commission of Inquiry established by the United Nations, between April and June 2011, Syrian security forces "carried out a wave of arrests against medical professionals in Damascus." In Aleppo, in June 2012, three medical professionals were arrested by Air Force Intelligence, and their burned bodies were found three days later (UN Human Rights, Office of the High Commissioner 2013).

One surgeon described the situation succinctly: "The events began in 2011 and I worked as an emergency physician. During the first attack of Deir ez-Zor the manager of the facility and I were arrested. We were arrested in August as soon as the military entered the city; we were detained for two days in Deir ez-Zor, then we were taken to Damascus and detained there for about eighteen days for questioning. We were accused of treating terrorists" (Interviewee 1023).

These and similar incidents throughout Syria suggest that already, within this first phase, the government had begun to consider health professionals a threat. Taking into account that a country's health system is a central tool for managing society and sustaining the population's productive energies in order to advance state goals, governments take it upon themselves to determine which health providers are legitimate, while criminalizing those that do not follow its edicts.[4] Not unlike the monopoly over the legitimate use of violence, in order to maintain control the state must preserve a *monopoly over the legitimate provision of health care.*[5] It is therefore not surprising that "83 percent of interviewees who were involved in the provision of medical aid to demonstrators in the first stages of the conflict reported they were subject to threats, including blacklisting, questioning, arrest, detention, torture, threatening of their family, expulsion from their job, and burning of their private practice."[6] As a precaution, doctors began adopting alternative means of communication with their networks, using pseudonyms when treating patients. Some even covered their faces so they could not be recognized. These doctors understood that by saving the lives of injured protesters, they had become, from the government's perspective, active agents of war and therefore targets for arrest and even assassination.

Phase 2: Health Providers as Enemies

During the second phase, the government lost its monopoly on violence as well as the means of coercion within Syria's sovereign territory (Munif 2020). At this point, there was an upsurge of diverse paramilitary organizations, and what had been a contiguous Syrian space was carved up and divided among the warring parties, producing significant territorial fragmentation (Dewachi et al. 2014). As the fighting continued, control over certain areas oscillated between different actors, and the borders demarcating each area were constantly changing. The degree of border permeability, which enabled or hindered the movement of people and goods across these internal frontiers, was also in flux and differed dramatically according to the area, the stage in the war, and the identity of belligerents controlling the territory in question.

These differences revealed themselves in MSF's interviews. A medical administrator from Idlib governorate described the internal borders of his area as hermetic—"as soon as you are in an opposition area you don't have any access to medical care on the regime side" (Interviewee 0008)—while a urologist from Quneitra explained that in the southern region, the borders were to some extent porous; there were secret access points, "or else we would have been smashed," he said with a laugh (Interviewee 1020).

As different areas were liberated from the government's control, health professionals aligned with the resistance took over governmental medical facilities and set up field hospitals, using them to offer care to both the civilian population and militants. A physician from Homs described the transition from the first to the second phase:

> At first, there were no fixed points. There were secret mobile points. Our work basically revolved around carrying mobile emergency bags in Homs neighborhoods . . . during the protests, people counted on mobile medical points. Then, they counted on private hospitals despite the security risk on the hospital and staff and the risk of patients wounded in protests getting arrested. . . . Afterwards, early 2012, I don't remember the exact date, military action started in the city and the countryside. Frankly, this gave us a great opportunity to use a big public hospital which was liberated by the military after it had been a detention and torture centre. . . . This military action enabled us to use the equipment available at the hospital and distribute it in Old Homs and its northern suburb areas. . . . We supported several regions, providing them with incubators, anaesthesia machine, and two ventilators, in addition to surgical drugs and tools for general and orthopaedic surgery. (Interviewee 2002)

The fragmentation of Syrian space unraveled the country's public health system. For months and sometimes years, certain populations were trapped within areas that did not have advanced tertiary care facilities, while other populations might have had access to some tertiary specialties but not to others. In a similar vein, the supply lines of medical goods were dramatically circumscribed, and even areas that did have tertiary facilities frequently found it difficult to provide necessary treatment due to a lack of medical equipment and medicine. A laboratory technician who became a medical equipment smuggler explained that "the ministry of health strictly forbids medicines and medical equipment to be transferred from regime-controlled areas to opposition-controlled areas." When asked how she managed to navigate checkpoints, she replied: "with money" (Interviewee 1026). A surgeon from Quneitra governorate noted that the "regime controls all access points and the entry and exit of all things, especially for medical and pharmaceutical items. Anything could be easier to introduce than medical items and equipment" (Interviewee 1020). The blockade on health care equipment was undoubtedly successful, with 86 percent of interviewees reporting that they lacked the necessary medication and medical supplies to do their jobs (MSF n.d.).

Nearly all interviewees intimated that provision of health care within the opposition-controlled areas was integral to the resistance's war effort, and indeed to the survival of the people whom the resistance represented. Without health professionals and functioning medical facilities, the resistance would have been rapidly defeated. It is therefore not necessarily surprising that, during this phase, healthcare providers became prime targets of the government.

The Counter-Terrorism Law adopted by the Syrian parliament in 2012 effectively criminalized the provision of aid to people living in opposition-controlled areas, legally rationalizing the arrest and prosecution of people involved in medical activities outside government-approved health structures (Human Rights Watch 2013; MSF n.d.). Hence, all health professionals practicing medicine outside areas controlled by the government as well as within government-controlled areas but not within sanctioned facilities were framed as enemies of the state. MSF found that even health professionals who worked in public and military hospitals were kept under permanent surveillance, while those who assisted people opposing the government were arrested and jailed. Some were eventually released, others died in detention, and the fate of many health workers is unknown to this day (Gladstone and Brown 2019).

Thus, in sharp contrast to the well-established and longstanding international legal norm that frames healthcare providers as neutral, medical professionals were deemed—and as the interviews suggest most of them considered themselves to be—partisan (Schmitt 2004). The government cast the opposition as legitimate targets of violence, using domestic criminal laws such as the Counter-Terrorism Law (Buzan and Hansen 2009). By framing the provision of health care as a key component of their enemies' war-making apparatus, the government securitized the opposition's medical field and thus paved the way for adopting emergency intervention against it (Buzan et al. 1998; Gordon 2014). This helps explain the criminalization of health professionals as well as the severe restrictions on the movement of medical goods.

Here we witness how domestic criminal law is invoked to facilitate the objectives of war. Human rights practitioners have criticized a similar process in Iraq, where the introduction and deployment of domestic anti-terrorism law was used to circumvent the protections international humanitarian law offers to belligerents (Houry 2019). What these practitioners failed to note is that international humanitarian law itself allows countries to invoke and use national criminal law within the framework of war, an issue I discuss below. But first, let's examine the third phase—which overlaps with the second phase—in which the Syrian government set out to completely destroy the medical field in opposition-controlled areas.

Phase 3: The Annihilation of Health Care

Médecins Sans Frontières's interviews with Syrian health professionals reveal how the medical field became a strategic target.[7] Physicians for Human Rights, USA, corroborated 595 attacks on at least 350 separate facilities and documented the killing of 923 medical personnel from March 2011 through February 2020. Although the actual number of attacks on medical units and staff was probably much higher, of the attacks examined by Physicians for Human Rights, 536, or 90 percent, were committed by the Syrian government and allied forces (Physicians for Human Rights 2020). What becomes clear from MSF's interviews is that the government identified the medical field as part of their enemies' war-making machine. As one general surgeon working in a city within the Damascus governorate put it, "The first thing the regime did after the city's liberation was to bomb the government hospital, which had regime-affiliated staff still working there" (Interviewee 2006). A general surgeon from Aleppo gave a sense of what this meant to the health professionals on the ground.

> While I was at Hospital One, the hospital was bombed more than twenty times. It was subject to direct bombing by a barrel or missile twice or three times per week, while in other situations a missile would hit five or ten meters away from the hospital. . . . All the buildings around the hospital were vacant, and no one would dare reside in its surroundings. . . . Once we were going to acquire a large basement in Aleppo to turn it into a hospital. . . . Yet the military parties which had facilities nearby objected that we would locate [our hospital] therein lest it would [increase the] risks to their military bases. The regime targeted the hospitals more than military points. (Interviewee 1028)

As a result of the bombings, health professionals in the opposition-controlled areas understood that they had to conceal their work. "The regime took revenge on the civilians by bombing every medical center established before [2011]," a nurse from Hama explained. "Consequently, they all went out of service. Civilians were thus deprived of medical services and this pushed us to establish this secret field hospital away from the region's center." When asked if by bombed centers she meant the governmental medical centers serving the regions, the nurse replied, "Yes, exactly. After the regime forces left, the first targets for the bombing were these centers" (Interviewee 2025). In a similar vein, a paramedic from Daraa recounted how "informants would tell officials the location of the medical points, and they would be bombed. As a result, we had to change locations several times" (Interviewee 2031).

To be sure, during this phase the Syrian government carried out indiscriminate bombing of entire areas, a practice enabled by a counter-terrorism logic that designated whole communities as hostile. Legally speaking, this is significant, because within a context of blanket bombings of civilian areas it is *predictable* that medical facilities will be destroyed, but it becomes difficult to prove that the government *intended* to target hospitals. And in international humanitarian law, intention is vital for demonstrating liability. Notwithstanding the distinction between predictable and intended consequences, the testimonies suggest that bombing of medical units became the norm, with 84 percent of interviewees working in opposition-controlled areas testifying that the health facilities in which they worked had been subject to shelling or bombing (MSF n.d.). At one point, according to those interviewed, even basements could not protect health professionals and their patients, and staff began devising methods to keep the locations of underground hospitals secret.

A dentist from Ghouta explained that fellow staff members established "entrances to the health facilities through tunnels which are five hundred or six hundred meters away from [the facilities themselves], so the Air Force would be unable to identify the hospital's specific location" (Interviewee 1016). In Latakia's Akrad mountains, health professionals established a hospital in a cave. It included an emergency room, an outpatient department, and a small maternity ward (Interviewee 0013). Slowly, in more and more provinces, the medical field was pushed underground. Yet even then, the government, which began receiving aerial assistance from the Russian Air Force in 2015, hunted the doctors and nurses down.[8] At a certain point, medical units receiving MSF assistance asked the humanitarian organization to stop sharing the GPS coordinates of their facilities with the Syrian government, a common practice used during war to help protect medical units from attack. MSF realized that instead of guaranteeing protection to these hospitals and staff, at times the coordinates enabled the government and its Russian ally to transform them into targets (Shaheen 2016). With the government disregarding the distinction between war-makers and health providers, strikes on hospitals and health professionals became a cornerstone in the military campaign to defeat its enemies.

In response to the devastation of health infrastructure in Syria, human rights and humanitarian organizations have invoked international human-itarian law to accuse the Syrian government of carrying out war crimes. The specific legal provisions dealing with health facilities and staff are in-formed by a norm that assumes medical units should be protected during armed conflict. The norm itself, however, like all other norms, is a histor-ical artifact and a site of struggle. It is produced and reinforced through repeated and ongoing citations, reiterations, and performances, and is, of course, subject to change over time (Butler 1990). Indeed, the idea of pro-viding protection to health providers is neither natural nor intrinsic to the function of the medical field and had to be produced by those who aspired to regulate the use of violence during war.

It is impossible to pinpoint exactly when the norm emerged. But we do know that after witnessing the horrors of war at Solferino, during the second War of Italian Independence, in 1859, Henri Dunant, a Swiss cit-izen who later helped found the International Committee of the Red Cross, spearheaded an effort to solidify a norm establishing protections to the wounded and sick as well as to health professionals during armed conflict (Dunant 2013; Nesiah 2016).[9] Perhaps his greatest achievement was his success in convincing the powerful countries of his time that taking care of the wounded and sick in the battlefield was in the interests of all war-ring parties (Moorehead 1999). To advance a moral norm that draws a di-rect link between human dignity and the protection of the medical field, Dunant and his co-conspirators persuaded the key actors that the norm would benefit all involved. On its own, the notion of human dignity appears to have been insufficient to "universalize" the norm, and therefore the idea of reciprocity was introduced, overtly interlacing morality with state in-terest (Kennedy 2008).

To do so Dunant framed the medical field as carrying out a humani-tarian mission that stood in sharp contrast to the destructive character of war-making. He described doctors, nurses, and medics as neutral. And the moral edict informing the medical field—"do no harm"—lent itself to this portrayal, given that it cuts across national boundaries. He then helped establish a charity organization of health-professional volunteers who would treat the wounded and sick, enabling him to cast the med-ical field as external to the war effort (Gross 2006). Ultimately, in the wake of these interventions, the norm offering medical units protections frames health care and war-making as if they were two independent fields, to be treated separately during armed conflict. Dunant's ability to universalize this interpretation lent the norm its legitimacy and authority (Moorehead 1999).

What we witnessed in Syria is not only the government's adoption of warfare strategies that ignore the legal protections offered to medical units, but also a different and more complex interpretation of the function of health care during war. The interviews MSF conducted vividly underscore that both war-makers and health providers are concerned with who may live and who must die (Foucault 2007; Mbembe 2003), though they operate in different ways, and their aims tend to differ as well. The operations of both fields are informed by the logic of "protecting" and "saving," and, not surprisingly, the analogy between war and health has a long history. As political scientist Colleen Bell points out, infectious and malignant diseases are a "threat" that medical experts are expected to attack, and if the patient survives, they are said to have "won the battle," while insurgents and rebels are often cast as a disease that needs to be eradicated in order to "save" the social body (Bell 2012). Indeed, killing in order to save is an integral part of the liberal war thesis (Dillon and Reid 2009).

There are, however, also significant differences between the two fields. War-makers are primarily concerned with saving the nation, protecting a territory from conquest, or defending a particular ideology, while health professionals are mostly involved with saving individual lives, even as epidimeology and public health are concerned with the social body as a whole. Perhaps the main difference between the two fields is their mode of action: states can legally exercise the right to kill during war and can often achieve the war's goal of saving and protecting through destruction and death (Goodman 2013),[10] while health professionals are obliged to act according to the moral edict "do no harm," and their actions focus on rescuing, healing, and sustaining life.

But the health professionals' descriptions of the unfolding events in Syria also clearly illustrate a profoundly paradoxical element to the dynamic between war-making and health care, given that the war-making apparatus actually depends on the medical field for its successful operation. In Syria, opposition-held areas trapped without medical services could not be sustained (Munif 2020). Indeed, health care is a necessary component of modern warfare not only because it provides care for wounded and sick combatants who may later return to take part in the fray, but also because it is essential for sustaining the social body and infrastructures of existence from which war-makers emanate and through which the war-making apparatus is maintained. It enables society to continue functioning before, during, and after wartime, which explains why states aim to maintain monopoly over the legitimate provision of health care. But just as health is integral to sovereign control, it is also a necessary component of those aiming to break the chains of control.

Médecins Sans Frontières's interviews suggest that without health professionals, war-makers may be able to liberate a territory, but they can neither protect nor sustain the population within that territory, intimating that the medical field is not antithetical or even external to the war effort. In a similar vein, political scientist Alison Howell has shown how military strategies have shaped medical science and vice versa, arguing that the two fields are symbiotically coproduced (Howell 2017).

Health providers are thus tied to war-makers in two primary ways. The logics of protecting and saving inform the operations of both fields, albeit in very different and at times opposing ways, and war-making *depends* on humanitarian work in order to function. If the norm aims to consti-tute the medical field as neutral and external to any war, MSF's interviews from Syria intimate that from the beginning, the Syrian government un-derstood and strove to position the medical field as inseparable from war. Saving the wounded protester was framed in relation to saving the nation, and because such an act was considered harmful to the nation, it had to be prevented. In addition, when health professionals have to hide, work in secret locations, use pseudonyms, and conceal their faces, they, too, as the interviews reveal, begin to understand their work as part of the war effort.

This had an immense impact on the activities of health professionals. A Syrian doctor, who was in the midst of training to become a pediatrician when the insurrection erupted, described how he discontinued his studies so he could practice medicine in a besieged region. "When we had first seen how they slaughtered children, we left," he said. "We wanted to assist with the revolution, and help people who are more in need here, and to be there for them. . . . I started working here in the clinics, in the liberated areas, and in the hospitals there" (Interviewee 1004). This doctor, like many other interviewees, perceived the humanitarian task of caring for the injured and sick as fundamental to the "revolution."

As the war unfolded and external forces entered the fray, the opposi-tion split into numerous factions. Consequently, any attempt to present the war in binary terms, as one between a government and a united op-position, would be misguided. The interviewees repeatedly referred to the complexity of the situation, underscoring at times that they were caught between the government's aerial onslaughts and the oppression on the ground by groups like the Islamic State. Such situations informed their decisions. Some chose to flee to other countries, while others stayed, un-derstanding their work as an act of multilayered resistance. Not surpris-ingly, many of the interviewees characterized themselves as partisan, using their medical knowledge to aid the opposition in its struggle against a corrupt authoritarian government.

Hence, the interviews indicate that both the Syrian government and health professionals themselves cast the medical field as a necessary component of the war effort, so much so that in the government's eyes, vanquishing their enemies' medical capabilities was essential for winning the war—as the actions of its security forces clearly reveal. This starkly contradicts one of the norm's basic assumptions that the medical field is impartial or external to war. The wide gap between the way the norm imagines the relation between health and war and the material way the relation has been performed in Syria ultimately weakens the norm providing medical units protection.[11]

INTERNATIONAL HUMANITARIAN LAW AND MEDICAL UNITS

One might say that the norm pertaining to health care in wartime focuses on what *ought* to be and aims to influence warring parties and health professionals to perform in a particular way by drawing a distinction between war-making and health care. By contrast, the Syrian government and those interviewed by MSF concentrate on what *is*—namely, the fact that on the ground, the two fields are intricately intertwined. The formal role of international humanitarian law is to help transform the *is* into the *ought*, and in our context to assert and then help produce a distinction between war-makers and health providers, while penalizing those who do not maintain the distinction.

An analysis of the legal provisions that articulate the specific protections offered to medical units during armed conflict lays bare that the law actually reflects and embodies the profound gap that exists between the norm, on the one hand, and how it is performed in conflict zones, on the other: The law sets out to produce a distinction between war-makers and health providers, but it is also acutely aware that the two fields overlap. Hence, one can trace a second gap—corresponding with the first one—within international humanitarian law itself. Before discussing this gap and the relevant legal provisions, however, it is important to note that the separation the norm constructs between war-makers and health care professionals corresponds with the more general and basic legal distinction between combatants and noncombatants.

At its core, international humanitarian law is based on a binary opposition between combatants, who are considered to be active war-makers who can be legitimately killed, and noncombatants, who are understood to be innocent and passive bystanders and are therefore offered a series of protections (Alexander 2007; Kinsella 2011). Hence, the civilian is the combatant's other, an inactive person trapped in the midst of war or under a belligerent occupation. Significantly, the four basic principles underlying humanitarian law—the principles of distinction, proportionality, military necessity, and humanity—are all based on the combatant/noncombatant divide. And this distinction provides the lens through which the law imagines war (Henckaerts et al. 2005).

Within this legal framework, and in the wake of the historical development of the norm dealing with medical units, health professionals and medical facilities came to be situated on the noncombatant side of the divide. The normative injunction to protect them emerges from their imagined role during war, from the idea that they do not participate in hostilities or in the war effort. Yet, as interviews with Syrian medical personnel underscore time and again, medical units are never passive in wartime, and it is also nearly impossible to imagine them as such.

Comparing the function of health professionals during armed conflict with a civilian who is, for example, aiding the war effort by working in a munitions factory elucidates the difference between noncombatants and health providers (Dinstein 2004). The spatial overlapping between the civilian, a protected person, and a munitions factory, a legitimate target, produces a legal threshold that renders the civilian a legitimate target. So long as the civilian does not enter the munitions factory, he or she preserves all the protections allocated to noncombatants. But the moment the civilian enters the factory, he or she can be legitimately killed. Civilians are defined as the absolute other of combatants and cross the line only when they assume a particular function that assists in the war effort, or when they occupy a legitimately targeted space. In the case of health professionals, by contrast, the legal threshold is embodied in the functionality of health care as a field. The threshold is always there, because their humanitarian mission helps secure the population's infrastructure of existence, which is, in turn, a constitutive and essential element of warmaking (Gordon and Perugini 2019). To exit or escape the threshold, health professionals must stop offering health care services and become civilians.

On the one hand, then, health providers are not combatants and do not participate in hostilities; on the other hand, they are an active, essential component of the war-making enterprise, because without them the infrastructure of existence and resistance would collapse. The medical field's function during armed conflict inevitably produces countless situations where health and war overlap, exposing why the very attempt to perceive medical facilities as external and neutral to conflicts inevitably creates tensions within the law. The legal provisions attempt to address these tensions by identifying and constructing medical units as protected sites and, simultaneously, as sites that can be attacked under certain conditions. Protection and exceptions to protections thus become the general schema characterizing the legal provisions involving medical units.

Protections and Exceptions

International humanitarian law appears to be at least partially aware of the liminal position of medical units in armed conflict and aims to resolve the matter by requiring health providers to mark themselves with insignia (Cauderay 1990). By introducing a distinguishing marker, the law itself produces the division between health providers and war-makers, and then calls upon belligerents to refrain from attacking medical units. There is undoubtedly much to praise about the effort to protect medical units, yet the law is, as mentioned, also acutely aware of the difficulty in sustaining a separation between health and war. To manage this tension, the law introduces a series of exceptions that aim to describe a number of situations in which health care and war-making noticeably overlap.

The schema of protection and exception to the protection is evident from the very first treaty that offered medical units protections, the 1864 First Geneva Convention for the Amelioration of the Condition of the Wounded in Armies in the Field. Article 1of the Convention notes that "ambulances and military hospitals shall be recognized as neutral, and as such, protected and respected by the belligerents as long as they accommodate wounded and sick" (First Geneva Convention 1864). The protections offered to health professionals are based on the recognition that they are neutral, a term that appears in five of the Convention's ten articles, thus reflecting and reinforcing the norm. Simultaneously, however, the protections are restricted to the act of accommodating the wounded and sick, intimating that other acts are not protected. Article 1 then adds an explicit exception, noting that "neutrality shall end if the said ambulances or hospitals should be held by a military force" (First Geneva Convention 1864).

Two issues emerge from the way the Convention formulates the protections offered to medical units. First, the Convention reiterates the norm's assumption that medical units and staff should remain neutral and, as such, must be perceived as external to the war-making machine. It is precisely this supposed neutrality and externality that helped convince countries to sign the Convention and offer health professionals protections (Moorehead 1999). Second, the schema of protection followed by an exception to the protection—a schema that accompanies international humanitarian law to this day—is both a result and a reflection of competing interpretations of health care's spatial position and function during war. This is apparent even within the most robust treaties regulating the deployment of violence during armed conflict: the 1977 Additional Protocols I and II to the Geneva Conventions. Additional Protocol I relates to international armed conflicts involving at least two countries, while Additional Protocol II is the first international treaty that applies solely to civil wars.[12] Because the Syrian war was a hybrid conflict, which first emerged as a civil war but rapidly assumed an international dimension following the intervention of numerous countries (Phillips 2016), both Protocols are relevant (Nebehay 2017).

When examining how the protection-exception schema is introduced in the provisions themselves, it is important to keep in mind that if protection symbolizes a form of restraint on violence, the exception signifies the unleashing of humanitarian violence. By humanitarian violence I mean the violence carried out in accordance with humanitarian law and supported by humanitarian organizations through their demand for legal accountability.[13] Precisely because violence is cast as humane—and therefore ethical and humanitarian—when it is used in a way that respects the legal provisions, it is significant to examine what the law says in relation to attacks on medical units.

The first clause of Article 12 of Additional Protocol I states, "Medical units shall be respected and protected at all times and shall not be the object of attack." But in the Article's fourth clause, this categorical injunction is qualified, and two exceptions are introduced: "Under no circumstances shall medical units be used in an attempt to shield military objectives from attack. Whenever possible, the Parties to the conflict shall ensure that medical units are so sited that attacks against military objectives do not imperil their safety."[14] There are, in other words, two situations in which a medical unit may lose its protections: If it shields combatants or harbors weapons it becomes susceptible to military strikes, and if it is located near a military target it is also susceptible to attacks (because it might be used to defend a munitions factory, military base, airfield, etc.).

Warring parties wishing to justify their attacks on medical units have historically invoked the latter provision, claiming that hospitals were deliberately placed near a legitimate target in order to shield it from attack (Gordon and Perugini 2019). The International Committee of the Red Cross (ICRC) adds in its commentary that the "deliberate siting of a medical unit in a position where it would impede an enemy attack" is sufficient for it to lose protection, provided the warring party abides by the principles of proportionality and military necessity (Pictet et al. 1987). Jonathan Whittall, director of MSF's analysis department, said in an interview that it would not be inconceivable for some belligerents to consider a hospital to be shielding if a wounded combatant were to use his cell phone to make a call from a hospital bed, because in their eyes the combatant could be directing military operations from the hospital. The shielding accusation, Whittall said, is a very slippery concept, and readily can be used by belligerents as an excuse for attacking medical units.[15] Therefore, following attacks on hospitals, such as the 2016 bombing of a cave hospital north of Hama, it is not surprising that the Russian deputy foreign minister, Gennady Gatilov, claimed that militants were using "so-called hospitals" as human shields (Francis 2016).

Article 13 introduces a third exception, stating that "the protection to which civilian medical units are entitled shall not cease *unless* they are used to commit, outside their humanitarian function, acts harmful to the enemy."[16] According to ICRC, "Such harmful acts would, for example, include the use of a hospital as a shelter for able-bodied combatants or fugitives, as an arms or ammunition dump, or as a military observation post; another instance would be the deliberate siting of a medical unit in a position where it would impede an enemy attack." What constitutes "harmful to the enemy" is in this way left open to interpretation and can be expanded dramatically by warring parties from the use of the medical facility to conceal combatants or arms to a patient-combatant making a call on his cell phone. ICRC's commentary fails to note that the notion of "humanitarian function" is not self-evident, and that warring parties also dispute the humanitarian nature of certain acts.

In a September 2019 press conference convened to speak about "numerous allegations of bombings of medical and other civilian facilities in Idlib," Russia's permanent representative to the United Nations, Vassily Nebenzia, discussed what he called "a whole new dimension of warfare, when modernly equipped, trained, and well-supplied non-state armed groups act as an effective party to armed conflict, but often manage to hide behind and invoke international humanitarian law."[17] Nebenzia described to his audience the following scenario:

> Now. You are a fighter on a battlefield. Suppose fighter jets are coming. You have a choice to hide in the nearest empty building or go into the one, which you reported as "de-conflicted," hoping that it would not be hit, since the UN shared its coordinates. What would you do? I leave this question open. Also, would you try to use this arrangement for your military advantage? Why not? The only thing, which can stop you, is the respect for Geneva Conventions, which directly

forbid to use civilian infrastructure to shield military objects, since that would compromise protected status (Additional Protocol I, Article 12). But would you expect Al-Nusra to respect the international humanitarian law? I would not.[18]

Thus, Russia's (and one can assume the Syrian government's) underlying assumption was that all medical units in areas controlled by the opposition were being used to commit acts harmful to the enemy. Hence, the exceptional situations—which according to international law strip medical units of their protections—were presented by the Russian diplomat as an a-priori rule. To preempt the charge that hospitals had been bombed in violation of international law, the diplomat explained at the beginning of the press conference that "the deliberate manipulation of information has become one of the most important weapons of this war."[19] The presumption is that the opposition will always deny that it was using medical units to advance its war efforts, and thus the debate is shifted from hospital bombings per se, to whether the bombing was legitimate given the legal exceptions.

Article 16 turns the focus to health professionals, stating that "under no circumstances shall any person be punished for having carried out medical activities compatible with medical ethics, regardless of the person benefiting therefrom."[20] The clause is clear that health professionals can treat enemy combatants and should not be punished for it. Yet, in Additional Protocol II, the one dealing with internal conflicts, this clause is also qualified, and an exception is introduced. After articulating in Article 10 an identical clause to Article 16 from Protocol I, Additional Protocol II inserts a third provision, stating that "the professional obligations of persons engaged in medical activities regarding information which they may acquire concerning the wounded and sick under their care shall, *subject to national law*, be respected"[21]

In its commentary, ICRC explains that national law refers "not only to the law in force at the start of the conflict, but also to any new legislation introduced and brought into force by a State after the start of the conflict. This legal situation, the result of a compromise, has its shortcomings in that it might endanger the special protection to which the wounded and sick should be entitled."[22] The Red Cross fails to note that extracting information from health professionals about their patients can be a pretense for many things, and may endanger the health professionals themselves and not just the patients. The Counter-Terrorism Law adopted by the Syrian parliament in 2012 is a case in point, given that it led to or at least facilitated numerous arrests, tortures, and disappearances of health professionals. More important, by giving precedence to national laws, including emergency laws introduced in the midst of war, the so-called compromise helps undo practically all the protections Additional Protocol II bestows on medical units.

The exceptions in these and other clauses indicate that the law accepts the foundational distinction between health care and war-making, but also presumes that this distinction is difficult to uphold. The law calls on parties to implement the distinction and to deploy warfare strategies that respect it, but at the same time introduces numerous exceptions, allowing belligerents to attack medical units in those instances in which the distinction is not upheld, and provided they abide by certain principles and conditions.[23]

Human rights and humanitarian organizations often criticize belligerents for violating the law. Yet, precisely in this context, it is important to recall the claim made by critical legal scholars, as well as by scholars carrying out critical legal feminist and race theory, that precisely because access to language is always mediated, every reading of the law is already an interpretation. Duncan Kennedy refers to interpretation as "legal work," characterizing it as a site of struggle where each interpretation is informed by the interpreter's ideological disposition and can advance different political and social goals. This, Kennedy emphasizes, does not mean that every interpretation goes, but it does follow that there are several valid interpretations to any legal provision (Kennedy 2008).

Clearly belligerents who bomb hospitals have a vested interest in interpreting the incident in a way that renders the exception applicable to the situation, while others may choose to highlight the protections. The difficulty arises because international law provides the attacking forces a large arsenal of exceptions with which to work. Considering that protections serve as a mechanism to fetter violence, while exceptions allow warring parties to unleash violence, it is vital to examine the relation between the two. As long as the exception is indeed exceptional, the law reasserts the primary distinction promulgated by the norm and restricts the deployment of violence. When the exception becomes the rule, however, the law itself ends up destabilizing the distinction advanced by the norm, while allowing the exercise of violence.

Elsewhere, Nicola Perugini and I have described the history of hospital bombings and documented the disturbing way different warring parties have managed to exploit the legal exceptions to justify attacks on medical units, accusing health professionals of failing to sustain a clear separation between life-enabling and war-making activities. We demonstrated that practically every time warring parties admitted they had bombed a hospital (and it was not a mistake), they invoked one of the legal exceptions to justify the act, while also chronicling the prevalence of such legal justifications throughout the history of warfare. We argued that the only way to reduce attacks on medical units was by offering them absolute and non-derogable protection, not unlike the ban on torture (Gordon and Perugini 2019). We did not, however, explain that the history of hospital bombings clearly illustrates how the exception actually has become the rule. The very laws aiming to reinforce the norm end up undermining it, helping to legitimize the deployment of violence against medical units.

LEGAL ADVOCACY

All of this brings us back to legal advocacy. The ultimate role of legal advocacy is to monitor and document behavior of both state and nonstate actors, and to try to influence them to abide by the edicts set out by humanitarian norms. Most human rights and humanitarian organizations consider the law to be the primary tool with which to achieve this, serving as the frame of reference for evaluating behavior while concurrently offering concrete guidelines on how actors should behave, as well as a series of penalties if they fail to comply. The law, in other words, is considered a norm-enhancing apparatus.

Yet, as I have demonstrated, the Syrian government not only defied the humanitarian norm that calls upon actors to protect medical units during armed conflict, but also appears to have specifically targeted medical units. And although in recent years most of the attacks on health facilities have taken place in Syria, medical units have been targeted in over twenty countries, according to the World Health Organization. Findings suggest that in 2016, a hospital was bombed, on average, every day and a half (WHO 2017), and in 2017 and 2018, a hospital was bombed every two days (WHO 2018). Granted that hospital bombing is not a new phenomenon (Durand and Boissier 1984), and that it is unclear whether historically there has been an increase in attacks on medical units, it is still important to inquire why the norm that the law is meant to protect and reinforce is so unstable.

As I have shown, the humanitarian norm is based on the separation between war-makers and health providers. Yet this separation is extremely difficult to sustain due to the function of health care and the particular role of health professionals in the war effort. I have suggested that not only the Syrian government, but also the health professionals on the ground, considered health workers to be partisan. A closer investigation of the law itself reveals that even as the law provides medical units with a series of protections that attempt to restrain violence, it also introduces several crucial exceptions, setting out conditions under which warring parties can legally unleash violence against health facilities and staff.

An analysis of the legal articles dealing with protections to medical units sheds light on the notion of sovereign exception. Although thinkers from Carl Schmitt to Georgio Agamben often have described the exception as a sovereign's decision to suspend the law (Schmitt 2005; Agamben 1998; Agamben 2005), a brief examination of international humanitarian law suggests that exceptions are an integral part of the law itself and a fundamental component of its ability to function. While Agamben claims that sovereign power can extricate itself entirely from the habitus of law, producing a violence that "can shed every relation to law," Stephen Humphreys has persuasively shown that even during states of emergency the sovereign operates within a juridical field (Agamben 2005, p. 59).[24]

My criticism is slightly different. To introduce the state of exception the sovereign does not need to suspend the law but to activate exceptions within the law. The whole spectrum of exceptions described above were introduced by sovereign states during the legal drafting process, and they readily can be used to counter the constraints within the law. This is probably most apparent in Additional Protocol II, which offers medical units protections only to assert the primacy of national laws and their ability to annul the protections. In Syria, this manifested itself through the adoption of the Counter-Terrorism Law of 2012. Hence, my interrogation suggests that exceptions inscribed *within* the laws of armed conflict and not necessarily the exception produced through the *suspension* of these laws renders the wounded, the sick, and the people who care for them killable. Indeed, the space between protections and exceptions is precisely the site where legal work is carried out.[25]

Such an analysis undoubtedly questions the liberal theoretical understanding dating back to Thomas Hobbes's social contract, which presumes that juridical processes can replace violence as a way of settling conflicts. This liberal storyline, which takes us from violence to law, as thinkers from Robert Cover to Judith Butler have noted, does not account for the violence of the law (Cover 1985; Butler 2020). International humanitarian law is actually straightforward when it comes to violence; rather than prohibiting violence, it regulates its deployment, providing concrete guidelines about who can be killed, what can be destroyed, and the repertoires of violence that can be legitimately used. Hence, the law enables and at times even facilitates violence, even though its primary role is to regulate it. With respect to hospitals, the law makes lofty claims about the importance of protecting the medical mission, but, as I have shown, it provides numerous exceptions that allow states to target medical units. Consequently, invoking the law to seek relief from violence is not necessarily the best strategy. In Butler's words, it may entail following a nightmarish circularity worthy of Kafka (Wade 2020).

My interrogation raises serious questions about the legalistic purview of many human rights and humanitarian organizations, which the legal historian Samuel Moyn has traced in his account of the change from an antiwar politics during the Vietnman War to an increasing emphasis on international law in the wake of Iraq's occupation (Moyn 2014). Referring to the extensive attacks on medical facilities in Syria, a Human Rights Watch researcher exclaimed: "We know hospitals are being attacked more and more, and in many cases they seem to be deliberate attacks. It's a violation of the law of war, and needs to be prosecuted as a war crime. We are calling for accountability" (Graham-Harrison 2016). In a similar vein, criticizing a January 2018 bombing of a hospital in Idlib, MSF's head of mission in North Syria claimed: "This latest incident demonstrates the brutality with which health care is coming under attack in Syria. The fact that this attack occurred on a facility while it was treating incoming patients is particularly egregious and a clear violation of international humanitarian law" (MSF 2018). Indeed, as the introduction to this chapter highlights, accountability for the violation of international humanitarian law has been the primary rallying cry for NGOs seeking justice in Syria.

My claim, however, is that insofar as legal exceptions are an integral part of the law, the law ultimately ends up weakening the humanitarian norm offering medical units protections, rather than reinforcing it. Thus, the more that humanitarian and human rights organizations invoke the law, and enter debates with governments that use the legal exceptions to justify strikes on hospitals, the more the imperative to protect medical units loses its authority and appeal. Put differently, through its numerous exceptions, the law itself sows doubt on the validity and solidity of the moral norm. This might help explain David Kennedy's claim that as "we use the [legal] discourse more, we believe it less" (Kennedy 2009).

This leads directly to my earlier assertion that only a complete ban on targeting medical units has any hope of reducing the violence. Once there is a ban, medical units cannot be legally bombed even when they overlap with war. And because health providers and war-makers will inevitably overlap in every armed conflict, the only way to stop the bombing is to introduce a ban. Although this recommendation does not address the urgency of developing new strategies to address the violence exerted against medical units—and although warring parties will still be able to provide no explanation, deny attribution, or maintain that the strike on the medical unit was unintended—if distinction between war-makers and medical units is the objective, then only a legal framework void of exceptions can reinforce the humanitarian norm.

ACKNOWLEDGMENTS

I would like to thank Penny Green, Craig Jones, Eva Nanopoulos, Catherine Rottenberg, and Jonathan Whittall for their comments and suggestions on an earlier draft.

NOTES

1. For how this framing persists see Michele Heisler, Elise Baker, and Donna McKay, "Attacks on Health Care in Syria—Normalizing Violations of Medical Neutrality?" *New England Journal of Medicine* 373, no. 26 (2015): 2489–91.
2. Consult reports on Syria under the country profiles of organizations such as Human Rights Watch, Amnesty International, Physicians for Human Rights, and numerous other organizations. One typical report is *Physicians for Human Rights, The Destruction of Hospitals—A Strategic Component in Regime Military Offensives*, May 2019, online at http://syriamap.phr.org/#/en/case-studies/5.
3. The questions revolved around five main topics: the obstacles and challenges interviewees faced to carry out their job and how those difficulties evolved over time; the coping mechanisms and strategies they developed to tackle those challenges; the consequences the conflict had on the medical care offered to patients; the conflict's impact on their professional and personal life; and their perception of external support. Médecins Sans Frontières, *Talking about Medical Assistance in Syria,* undated draft.
4. On the notion of biopolitics see Michel Foucault, *Society Must Be Defended: Lectures at the Collège de France, 1975–1976.* Edited by Mauro Bertani and Alexandro Fontana. Translated by David Macey. Macmillan, 2003.
5. On the state's monopoly of legitimate violence see Max Weber, David S. Owen, and Tracy B. Strong, *The Vocation Lectures.* Hackett Publishing, 2004.
6. About one out of three interviewees was arrested, half of whom reported they were tortured in prison. Médecins Sans Frontières, *Talking about Medical Assistance in Syria,* undated draft.
7. For in-depth news reporting on hospital bombings see Malachy Browne, Christiaan Triebert, Evan Hill, Whitney Hurst, Gabriel Gianordoli, and Dmitriy Khavin, "Hospitals and Schools Are Being Bombed in Syria, A U.N. Inquiry Is Limited. We Took a Deeper Look," *New York Times*, December 31, 2019 and Whitney Hurst and Rick Gladstone, "U.N. Query on Syria Hospital Bombings May Be Undermined by Russia Pressure, Limited Scope," *New York Times*, November 14, 2019.
8. According to Airwars, the Russians carried out at least 39,000 airstrikes from 2015 to 2018. See Russian Military in Syria online at https://airwars.org/ conflict/russian-military-in-syria/; see also Browne et al., "Hospitals and Schools Are Being Bombed in Syria," *New York Times, 2019.*

9. At the time, Dunant also was engaged in a series of business ventures in the French colonies, including with Compagnie Genevoise des Colonies de Sétif (The Geneva Company of Colonies of Setif), and was entrusted with securing a land grant in Algeria, and facilitating European settlers access to local resources.
10. On the productive capacity of war see Tarak Barkawi, "From War to Security: Security Studies, the Wider Agenda and the Fate of the Study of War," *Millennium—Journal of International Studies* 39, no. 3 (2011): 701–16.
11. For an analysis of the gap between the norm and international humanitarian law see Cherif M. Bassiouni, "The Normative Framework of International Humanitarian Law: Overlaps, Gaps, and Ambiguities." *International Law Studies* 75, no. 1 (2000): 23.
12. Protocol Additional to the Geneva Conventions of 12 August 1949, Relating to the Protection of Victims of International Armed Conflicts, June 8, 1977, 1125 U.N.T.S. 3 (here thereafter Additional Protocol I). Protocol Additional to the Geneva Conventions of 12 August 1949, and Relating to the Protection of Victims of Non-International Armed Conflicts [hereinafter 1977 Protocol II], Dec. 12, 1977, U.N. Doc. N32/144 (here thereafter Additional Protocol II).
13. For more on the relation between humanitarianism and violence see Costas Douzinas, "The Many Faces of Humanitarianism" *Parrhesia* 2, no. 1 (2007): 28.
14. Additional Protocol I.
15. E-mail interview with Jonathan Whittall, March 26, 2018.
16. Additional Protocol I.
17. Permanent Representative of the Russian Federation at the United Nations, "Press-Conference by Permanent Representative Vassily Nebenzia on "Reports over Alleged Attacks on Healthcare in North-West Syria," September 16, 2019 online at https://russiaun.ru/en/news/press_conference1609
18. Permanent Representative of the Russian Federation at the United Nations, "Press-Conference," September 16, 2019.
19. Permanent Representative of the Russian Federation at the United Nations, "Press-Conference," September 16, 2019.
20. Additional Protocol II.
21. Additional Protocol II. Italics added.
22. Geneva Conventions of 1949 and Additional Protocols, and their Commentaries, Protocol Additional to the Geneva Conventions of 12 August 1949, and relating to the Protection of Victims of Non-International Armed Conflicts (Protocol II), 8 June 1977. Commentary of 1987 General protection of medical duties, paragraph 4699 online at https://ihl-databases.icrc.org/applic/ihl/ihl.nsf/Comment.xsp?action=openDocument&documentId=1E86B663DA082F6AC125 63CD0043A78E.
23. I discuss the precise conditions in Gordon and Perugini, "'Hospital Shields' and the Limits of International Law," 2019.
24. For a criticism of Agamben, which shows how even in a state of emergency the law is not suspended see Stephen Humphreys, "Legalizing Lawlessness: On Giorgio Agamben's *State of Exception*," *European Journal of International Law* 17, Issue 3 (1 June 2006): 677–87. https://doi.org/10.1093/ejil/chl020.
25. On the kind of legal work see Craig Jones, *The War Lawyers: The United States, Israel and Juridical Warfare*. London and New York: Oxford University Press, 2020.

REFERENCES

Agamben, Giorgio. 1998. *Homo Sacer: Sovereign Power and Bare Life*. Redwood City, CA: Stanford University Press.

Agamben, Giorgio. 2005. *State of Exception*. Chicago: University of Chicago Press.

Alexander, Amanda. 2007. "The Genesis of the Civilian." *Leiden Journal of International Law 20* (2)): 359–76.

Bell, Colleen. 2012. "War and the Allegory of Medical Intervention: Why Metaphors Matter." *International Political Sociology 6* (3): 325–28.

Berkovitch, Nitza and Neve Gordon, "The Political Economy of Transnational Regimes: The Case of Human Rights." *International Studies Quarterly 52* (4): 881–904.

Butler, Judith. 1990. *Gender Trouble: Feminism and the Subversion of Identity*. New York: Routledge.

Butler, Judith. 2020. *The Force of Nonviolence: The Ethical in the Political*. London: Verso Books.

Buzan, Barry, Ole Wæver, and Jaap de Wilde. 1998. *Security: A New Framework for Analysis*. Boulder, Colorado: Lynne Rienner Publishers.

Buzan, Barry and Lene Hansen. 2009. *The Evolution of International Security Studies*. Cambridge: Cambridge University Press.

Cauderay, Gerald C. 1990. "Visibility of the Distinctive Emblem on Medical Establishments, Units, and Transports." *International Review of the Red Cross Archive 30* (277): 295–321.

Cover, Robert M. 1985 "Violence and the Word." *Yale Law Journal 95*: 1601.

Dewachi, Omar, Mac Skelton, Vinh-Kim Nguyen, Fouad M. Fouad, Ghassan Abu Sitta, Zeina Maasri, and Rita Giacaman. 2014. "Changing Therapeutic Geographies of the Iraqi and Syrian Wars." *Lancet 383* (9915): 449–57.

Dillon, Michael and Julian Reid. 2009. *The Liberal Way of War: Killing to Make Life Live*. London: Routledge.

Dinstein, Yoram. 2004. *The Conduct of Hostilities under the Law of International Armed Conflict*. Cambridge: Cambridge University Press.

Douzinas, Costas. 2007. *Human Right s and Empire: The Political Philosophy of Cosmopolitanism*. London: Routledge.

Drumbl, Mark A. 2007. *Atrocity, Punishment, and International Law*. Cambridge: Cambridge University Press.

Dunant, Henri. 2013. *A Memory of Solferino*. Cambridge, UK: Ravenio Books.

Durand, André and Pierre Boissier. 1984. *From Sarajevo to Hiroshima: History of the International Committee of the Red Cross*. Geneva: Henry Dunant Institute.

First Geneva Convention, "Convention for the Amelioration of the Condition of the Wounded in Armies in the Field" (1864). https://ihl-databases.icrc.org/ihl/INTRO/120?OpenDocument

Foucault, Michel. 2007. *Security, Territory, Population: Lectures at the Collège de France 1977–1978*. London: Palgrave McMillan.

Francis, Ellen. "Even in a Bunker under a Mountain, Syrian Hospital Knocked Out by Strikes," *Reuters*, October 3, 2016. https://www.reuters.com/article/us-mideast-crisis-syria-hospital/even-in-a-bunker-under-a-mountain-syrian-hospital-knocked-out-by-strikes-idUSKCN1231RQ.

Gladstone, Rick and Malachy Browne. "Where Doctors are Criminals," *New York Times*, December 21, 2019.

Goodman, Ryan. 2013. "The Power to Kill or Capture Enemy Combatants," *European Journal of International Law* 24 (30): 819–53. https://doi.org/10.1093/ejil/cht048.

Gordon, Neve. 2014. "Human Rights as a Security Threat: Lawfare and the Campaign against Human Rights NGOs." *Law & Society Review* 48 (2): 311–44.

Gordon, Neve and Nicola Perugini. 2019. "'Hospital Shields' and the Limits of International Law." *European Journal of International Law* 30 (2): 439–63.

Graham-Harrison, Emma. "Aleppo Hospitals Are Latest Casualty in Attacks by the Syrian Regime," *The Guardian*, September 28, 2016.

Gross, Michael L. 2006. *Bioethics and Armed Conflict: Moral Dilemmas of Medicine and War*. Cambridge, MA: MIT Press.

Henckaerts, Jean-Marie, Louise Doswald-Beck, and Carolin Alvermann, Eds. 2005. *Customary International Humanitarian Law*. Cambridge: Cambridge University Press.

Howell, Alison. 2017. "Neuroscience and War: Human Enhancement, Soldier Rehabilitation, and the Ethical Limits of Dual-Use Frameworks," *Millennium—Journal of International Studies* 45 (2): 133–50.

Hopgood, Stephen. 2013. *The Endtimes of Human Rights*. Ithaca, NY: Cornell University Press.

Houry, Nadim. 2019. "Bringing ISIS to Justice: Running Out of Time?" *Just Security*. https://www.justsecurity.org/62483/bringing-isis-justice-running-time/.

Human Rights Watch. 2013. "Syria: Counterterrorism Court Used to Stifle Dissent." https://www.hrw.org/news/2013/06/25/syria-counterterrorism-court-used-stifle-dissent

Kennedy, David. 2005. *The Dark Sides of Virtue: Reassessing International Humanitarianism*. Princeton, NJ: Princeton University Press.

Kennedy, David. 2009. *Of War and Law*. Princeton, NJ: Princeton University Press.

Kennedy, Duncan. 2008. "A Left/Phenomenological Alternative to the Hart/Kelsen Theory of Legal Interpretation." In *Legal Reasoning: Collected Essays*, edited by Duncan Kennedy. Aurora, CO: Davies Group.

Kinsella, Helen M. 2011. *The Image Before the Weapon: A Critical History of the Distinction between Combatant and Civilian*. Ithaca, NY: Cornell University Press.

Marks, Susan. 2011. "Human Rights and Root Causes." *The Modern Law Review* 74 (1): 57–78.

Mbembe, Achille. 2003. "Necropolitics." *Public Culture* 15: 11.

Médecins Sans Frontières. "MSF-supported hospital in Idlib closed after damage from airstrikes" MSF Statement, January 29, 2018. https://www.msf.org/syria-msf-supported-hospital-idlib-closed-after-damage-airstrikes.

Médecins Sans Frontières. *Talking about Medical Assistance in Syria*, undated draft.

Meron, Theodor. 1989. *Human Rights and Humanitarian Norms as Customary Law*. Oxford: Clarendon Press.

Moorehead, Caroline. 1999. *Dunant's Dream: War, Switzerland and History of the Red Cross*. New York: Harper Collins Publishers.

Moyn, Samuel. 2014. "From Antiwar Politics to Antitorture Politics." *Stanford Scholarship Online*. https://papers.ssrn.com/sol3/papers.cfm?abstract_id=1966231

Munif, Yasser. 2020. *The Syrian Revolution: Between the Politics of Life and the Geopolitics of Death*. London: Pluto.

Mutua, Makau. 2001. "Savages, Victims, and Saviors: The Metaphor of Human Rights." *Harvard International Law Journal* 42: 201.

Nagy, Rosemary. 2008. "Transitional Justice as Global Project: Critical Reflections." *Third World Quarterly* 29 (2): 275–89.

Nebehay, Stephanie. "Situation in Syria Constitutes International Armed Conflict— Red Cross," *Reuters*, April 7, 2017.

Nesiah, Vasuki. 2016. "Human Shields/Human Crosshairs: Colonial Legacies and Contemporary Wars." *AJIL Unbound 110*: 323–28.

Pearlman, Wendy R. 2017. *We Crossed a Bridge and It Trembled: Voices from Syria.* New York: Custom House.

Perugini, Nicola and Neve Gordon. 2015. *The Human Right to Dominate.* London and New York: Oxford University Press.

Phillips, Christopher. 2016. *The Battle for Syria: International Rivalry in the New Middle East.* New Haven, CT: Yale University Press.

Physicians for Human Rights. 2019. "*The Syrian Conflict: Eight Years of Devastation and Destruction of the Health System.*" https://phr.org/wp-content/uploads/2019/03/PHR-Syria-2019-Fact-Sheet.pdf

Physicians for Human Rights. 2020. "Findings of Attacks on Health Care in Syria. http://syriamap.phr.org/#/en/findings.

Hans-Peter Gasser, Sylvie-So Junod,·Claude Pilloud, Jean de Preux, Yves Sandoz, Christophe Swinarski, Claude F. Wenger, Bruno Zimmermann. 1987. *Commentary on the Additional Protocols: of 8 June 1977 to the Geneva Conventions of 12 August 1949.*

Safeguarding Health in Conflict, *Syria.* 2018. https://www.safeguardinghealth.org/syria

Schmitt, Carl. 2004. *Theory of the Partisan: A Commentary/Remark on the Concept of the Political.* New York: Telos Press.

Schmitt, Carl. 2005. *Political Theology: Four Chapters on the Concept of Sovereignty.* Chicago: University of Chicago Press.

Shaheen, Kareem. "MSF Stops Sharing Syria Hospital Locations after 'Deliberate' Attacks," *The Guardian*, February 18, 2016.

United Nations Human Rights, Office of the High Commissioner, "Assault on Medical Care: A Distinct and Chilling Reality of the Civil War in Syria," October 2013. https://www.ohchr.org/EN/NewsEvents/Pages/AssaultOnMedicalCare.aspx.

Wade, Francis. "Judith Butler on the Violence of Neglect Amid a Health Crisis: A conversation with the theorist about her new book, *The Force of Nonviolence*, and the need for global solidarity in the pandemic world," *The Nation*, May 13, 2020.

Wedeen, Lisa. 2019. *Authoritarian Apprehensions: Ideology, Judgment, and Mourning in Syria.* Chicago: University of Chicago Press.

WHO (World Health Organization). Attacks on Health Care Dashboard, Reporting Period: 1 January to 31 December 2016. https://www.who.int/emergencies/attacks-on-health-care/attacks_dashboard_2016_updated-June2017.pdf?ua=1.

WHO (World Health Organization). Attacks on Health Care Dashboard, Reporting Period: 1 January to 31 December 2017. https://www.who.int/emergencies/attacks-on-health-care/dashboard2017-full.pdf?ua=1. World Health Organization, Attacks on Health Care Dashboard, Reporting period: 1 January to 31 December 2018, online at https://www.who.int/emergencies/attacks-on-health-care/attacks-dashboard-2018-full.pdf?ua=1.

CHAPTER 4

When Perceptions and Aspirations Clash

Humanitarianism in Syria's Neighboring States

DAWN CHATTY

THE MAKING AND UNMAKING OF A REFUGE STATE IN SYRIA

Twice in modern history Syria and its peoples have been at the epicenter of massive displacement. In the seventy years between 1850 and 1920, Syria received between three and four million forced migrants from the contested borderlands with the Imperial Russian and Ottoman Empires. At the close of the Crimean War (1853–1856), and the Ottoman–Russian Wars of the 1860s and 1880s, more than three million forced migrants from the Crimea, the Caucasus, and the Balkans entered the Ottoman provinces of Anatolia; many continued on their journeys to the Arab regions of Bilad al-Sham (Greater Syria). The Ottoman administration, in the aftermath of what many historians labeled the first genocide in modern history, established a special commission to address the needs of these forcibly displaced Tatars, Circassians, Chechens, Abkhazians, Abazas, and other related ethnic groups from the Trans-Caucasus region. This "refugee" commission, the *Muhacirin Komisyonu*—the first of its kind in contemporary European history—set out generous terms for resettlement, granting the migrants some freedom of choice along the sparsely settled agricultural lands of Greater Syria. It offered incoming forced migrants agricultural land, draft animals, seeds, and support in the form of tax relief for a

Dawn Chatty, *When Perceptions and Aspirations Clash* In: *Everybody's War.* Edited by: Jehan Bseiso,
Michiel Hofman, and Jonathan Whittall, Oxford University Press. © Médecins Sans Frontières 2021.
DOI: 10.1093/oso/9780197514641.003.0005

decade, as well as exemptions from military service (Chatty 2010). The goal was to help these settlers become self-sufficient in as short a time as possible. Integration into numerous ethnically mixed settlements of Greater Syria was encouraged, to promote and preserve the cosmopolitan, convivial nature of urban and rural communities in the late Ottoman Empire.

At the end of World War I, as many as 500,000 Armenians found refuge in Syria, settling among their coreligionists in Aleppo, Damascus, and Beirut. When the modern Republic of Turkey was established, in 1923, 10,000 Kurds from Turkey fled across the border into Syria, to escape the forced secularism of Mustafa Kemal Atatürk's new Turkey. The Inter-War French mandate over Syria saw a continuation of these processes, with tens of thousands of Assyrian Christians from Iraq entering the country in the 1930s, seeking asylum and safety after the Semele massacres of 1933. All these forced migrants were granted citizenship in the new Syrian state. In the late 1940s, Syria was again a safe harbor—this time for over 100,000 Palestinians fleeing the ethnic cleansing of the "Nakba" during the creation of the State of Israel. It is hardly an exaggeration to say that the modern "truncated" Syrian state, carved out of Greater Syria by the League of Nations in 1920 and granted full independence in 1946, was a place of refuge for hundreds of thousands, if not millions, of ethnoreligious minorities uprooted from their homelands near and far as a result of war, arbitrary lines drawn across maps, and ethnosectarian strife.

These newcomers to Syria—following on from the local and regional administrative structures first instituted by the Ottomans in their Tanzimat, or reform, period—formed strong horizontal ties to other coreligionists and ethnic groups scattered around the region. Armenians, for example, looked to their Apostolic Church for social and religious guidance, and recognized their ties with other Armenians dispersed around the country and into their frontier zones. Borders marked out in the 1920s and modified in the late 1930s cut across ethnoreligious communities who largely maintained cross-border relationships with their social groups in Turkey, Lebanon, Jordan, and Iraq (see Figure 4.1a–g and Table 4.1).

The second half of the twentieth century saw another wave of exodus into Syria. Many thousands of Palestinians sought refuge in the country following the Six-Day War of 1967, as did hundreds of thousands of Lebanese fleeing their civil war (1975–1989) and, increasingly, Iraqis fleeing the ever more despotic regime in their country. Even in the early twenty-first century, Syria admitted over a million Iraqi refugees into the country, hosting them as "temporary guests" and brother Arabs. As long as they and other refugees from Afghanistan, Sudan, Somalia, and Eritrea conducted their business without crossing any red lines or raising their heads above the

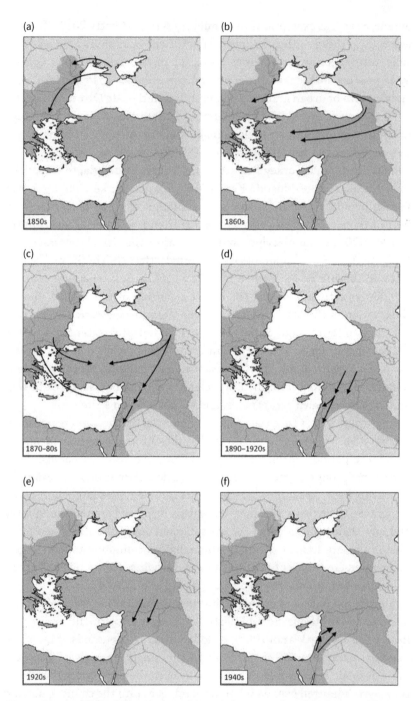

(a) 1850s

(b) 1860s

(c) 1870–80s

(d) 1890–1920s

(e) 1920s

(f) 1940s

Figure 4.1. a–g Maps of nineteenth- and twentieth-century forced migrations to Syria.
Source: Dawn Chatty.

(g)

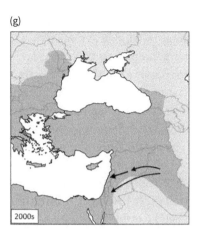

2000s

Figure 4.1 *Continued*

Table 4.1 KEY TO FIGURE 4.1 A–G

Key	
1860–1920s	Muslim Tatars, Circassians and other Caucasian groups
1890–1920s	Armenians
1920s	Kurds
1930s	Assyrians
1940s	Palestinians
2000s	Iraqis

parapet, they were tolerated by the Syrian Baathi state. The Arab and Syrian institution of hospitality and refuge meant that, until 2011, the West and its humanitarian aid architecture were relieved from having to deal with any mass influx of Iraqi or other refugees from the Arab world into Europe.

Then, a decade into the twenty-first century, Syria disintegrated into extreme violence, triggering a displacement crisis of massive proportions. The speed with which the country emptied of nearly 50 percent of its population shocked the world and left Western humanitarian aid agencies in turmoil, as they struggled to respond to the growing crisis on Syria's borders. Each country bordering Syria responded differently to this complex emergency, depending on its history of forced migration and colonial border elaborations. Turkey rushed to set up its own refugee camps—temporary towns—for the most vulnerable groups, but generally supported the self-settlement of Syrians among those they were closely tied to. Lebanon refused to allow the international humanitarian aid architecture to set up formal refugee camps, relying on Syrians who habitually worked in the country to develop an organic process of shelter. And Jordan, publicly open-armed, prevaricated for nearly a year before insisting on the establishment of a massive United Nations refugee camp at Za'tari. Turkey and Lebanon have permitted Syrians to enter as temporary "guests." Since 2014, Jordan has refouled, or returned, some Syrians to their country, contrary to international norms. And since 2016, Turkey and Lebanon have begun to do the same, under the banner of "voluntary" return.

It is significant to remember that Lebanon and Jordan have not signed onto the United Nations' 1951 Refugee Convention, which sets out the principles and responsibilities by which states ought to provide protection and asylum for those deemed to fit the definition of "refugee," according to the 1951 Statutes and the 1967 Protocol. And although Turkey has signed the 1951 Convention, it has reserved its interpretation of the agreement to apply only to Europeans seeking refuge in Turkey. The United Nations estimates that 60 to 70 percent of the Syrian refugee flow across international borders are self-settling in cities, towns, and villages where they have social networks. In Turkey, most refugees are clustered in the southern region of the country bordering Syria, where they have historically strong social and economic ties. Turkey also permitted, until very recently, circular movement of displaced Syrians back and forth between Syria and Turkey—for example, to check on property or elderly family members who refused to move. Despite a general rejection of encampment among those Syrians fleeing, some 20 to 25 percent of the Syrian refugee flow was, until recently, directed into camps. In Lebanon, informal tented settlements—often based on preexisting relationships with middlemen or "gang masters" who managed the hiring and wage structure of agricultural workers—are proliferating, with an accompanying re-emergence of patron-client relationships overcoming the more participatory and transparent management espoused by the international humanitarian aid architecture. In Jordan, where 80 to 85 percent of Syrians are self-settled, mainly in the northern part of the country bordering Syria, those found to be illegally working—working without work permits—are arrested. They are then "deported" into the UN-managed refugee camps of Za'tari or Azraq, from which there is no escape, other than paying to be sponsored by a Jordanian or to be smuggled out, after which they re-enter the liminal state of irregular status and work without permits (see Figure 4.2).

Turkey, Lebanon, and Jordan have established a variety of temporary measures to deal with the mass influx of displaced Syrians—but in no case have displaced Syrians or local host communities been consulted about

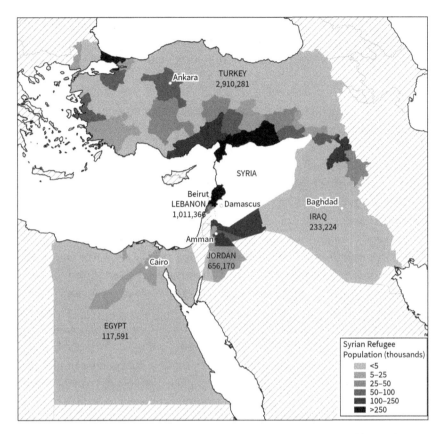

Figure 4.2. Map of displaced Syrians—self-settled and in camps—in neighboring hosting countries (November 2017).
Source: UNHCR MENA Office, Amman.

their aspirations or preferences. Discrepancies between what is wanted and what is needed by the involved parties and what is actually provided have rapidly become visible, and tensions and protests have quickly emerged among host communities, displaced Syrians, and humanitarian policymakers. This situation is unsustainable and threatens to test the Western humanitarian aid architecture's preferred solution of regionally containing the crisis (for instance, via "The EU Facility for Refugees in Turkey," usually referred to as the EU-Turkey deal, which pays Turkey to prevent Syrians from leaving Turkey to cross into Europe in exchange for easing of visa restrictions on Turkish citizens into the European Union). Without significant changes in policy and practice throughout the region, Syria's forced migrants will continue to flee in search of safety for their families and protection—temporary protection—elsewhere. Unable to work and provide their children with quality education, they will continue to move on, risking their lives in dangerous sea crossings and exhausting land marches led by smugglers. And those unable to move on continue to be targeted by state apparatus for "voluntary" return to an unsafe Syria.

REGIONAL CONTAINMENT POLICY: A CLASH OF PERCEPTIONS AND ASPIRATIONS

This research sets out to understand the disparity in perceptions, aspirations, and behavior of refugees from Syria, members of host communities, and aid practitioners in Turkey, Jordan, and Lebanon. It also seeks to identify what measures, if any, are regarded as important by these groups for future return and reintegration in Syria when conditions permit.

The methodology and methods applied are based on a multisited, twelve-month qualitative and participatory study conducted between October 2014 and September 2015 in Turkey, Lebanon, and Jordan (Amman and Irbid). I conducted interviews in Arabic and English, and interpretation was required only in Turkey when interviewing members of local Turkish-speaking communities hosting refugees from Syria. Once the initial key informants were selected, using a purposive sampling approach, a snowballing technique was employed to identify further interview participants, keeping an eye on representativeness in terms of gender, class, education, ethnicity, and place of origin. A participant observation strategy also defined this study.

In addition, the study initiated a consultative engagement between aid practitioners, representatives of hosting communities, and refugees. It commenced with in-country recruitment of researchers in collaboration with facilitating research institutions: the Swedish Research Institute in Istanbul, in Turkey; the American University of Beirut, in Lebanon; and the Council for British Research in the Levant, in Jordan. Fieldwork was divided into three one-month phases in each country: October 2014 in Istanbul, Ankara, and Gaziantep, Turkey; December 2014 in Beirut and the Bekaa Valley, Lebanon; and February 2015 in Amman and Irbid, Jordan. Each field trip included exploratory informal and focused discussions as well as semistructured interviews with international and national aid practitioners, self-settled refugees, and host community members, as well as refugees in camps in Turkey and Jordan.

A follow-up period of fieldwork in Lebanon, Jordan, and Turkey took place in April and May 2015, to collect further interviews related to the coping strategies of displaced Syrian families in Amman, Beirut, and Istanbul. These in-depth, one-on-one interviews and group discussions focused on the ways in which Syrian families were managing their relations with host communities and their interactions with the international aid sector.

LEBANON

Many Syrians in Lebanon displaced by the conflict in Syria do not feel that they are refugees. Some have strong kinship ties dating to the creation of "Greater Lebanon" during the Inter-War French mandate of 1920–1943, when the Bekaa Valley and Tripoli in the north were taken from Syria and added to the new Lebanese state. Hence many families have kinship relations that cross the Lebanon-Syria divide. Despite these ties, Syrians in Lebanon are aware of a growing level of social discrimination, especially in Beirut. Wealthy and middle-class Syrians are less affected by this discrimination and have been active in setting up associations to help the poorer members of the displaced Syrian community. Despite their efforts at solidarity, they express fear that the Lebanese population increasingly associates them with a rise in criminality, as regularly articulated in the Lebanese press. Of the nearly one thousand municipalities in the country, forty were quick to impose curfews on Syrians from dusk to dawn, making it difficult for some family heads of household to work and remain self-sufficient (Chatty 2017).

The Lebanese government's response to the Syrian crisis has been minimal and contradictory, reflecting the nature of the state and its consociational Parliament. The Lebanese government is made up of numerous ethno-religious political parties, many of which have constitutionally guaranteed seats in parliament. Furthering this fractured legislature is the strength of two political coalitions that emerged after the assassination of Prime Minister Rafiq Hariri in 2005: the US- and Saudi-backed March 14 Alliance, united by its anti-Syrian stance; and the March 8 Alliance, backed by Iran, which is strongly pro-Syrian. Between 2014 and 2016, Lebanon had no effective government. Only in October 2016 was the twenty-nine-month political deadlock broken, with the election of President Michel Aoun, who later named Saad Hariri as prime minister.

This complex government structure has meant that the international humanitarian architecture has been unable to move effectively in Lebanon. Early in the crisis, the government refused all efforts to establish refugee camps in the country, perhaps fearing that such a concentration of displaced Syrians might result in the same kind of extreme violence directed at Palestinian refugee camps during the Lebanese Civil War. With no opportunity to set up camps, the United Nations High Commissioner for Refugees (UNHCR) took to registering Syrians, as a step in the direction of providing protection and distributing cash assistance and other forms of aid to the most vulnerable. But in 2015, the Lebanese authorities requested that all United Nations refugee registration be stopped; the number of displaced Syrians in the country had exceeded one million, nearly a quarter of the national population. With little if any national assistance available to the displaced Syrians, international organizations and non-governmental organizations (NGOs)—international and national—had to step in and find creative ways to reach the displaced.

Most Syrians in Lebanon were not new to the country but had been working for years in the construction and agriculture sectors of the economy. During economic growth periods, the country had nearly five hundred thousand Syrian seasonal workers. The armed conflict and lack of reconstruction in Syria meant that many of the Syrian workers' wives and children fled the country to join husbands and fathers who'd already been working in Lebanon for some time. Their movements were largely progressive and in stages: they first arrived in Akkar or the Wadi Khaled region of northern Lebanon, and gradually made their way to join men working in the Bekaa Valley, Tripoli, and Beirut. For Syrians legally in Lebanon, these reunions with wives and children created great anxiety. Those with jobs feared losing them once it was known their families had joined them, contributing to feelings of fear, distress, and isolation. One Syrian woman described her family's situation as follows:

> My husband came to Lebanon a long time ago, even before the war in Syria. He used to come over since he was seventeen, therefore he knows Lebanon very well. He used to come and go, stay for a while [working as a carpenter], and then go back to Syria. In 2011 he was in Lebanon; then the situation was very bad in Syria, so I came to Lebanon . . . my husband had a job, and we stayed at his boss's house. Back then I could not go back to Hama. My husband had no intention of bringing me to Lebanon; for him it was settled that he worked in Lebanon and I stayed in Syria. But after all the explosions in Hama, I could not protect my kids. I decided to come and stay in Lebanon. My husband is always afraid he might be fired [if the children get into any trouble]. (interview with Reem, Beirut, 2014)

Illegal curfews in over forty municipalities (spread out over Lebanon's 1,550 villages) have meant that in these areas many Syrian men are afraid to go out at night, to work overtime, or to mix in any way with the Lebanese population. For many skilled and unskilled Syrians, these curfews have meant that older children and adolescents have been pulled out of whatever schooling they had been entered into in order to work during daylight hours with their fathers. As one woman explained:

> My son should be in ninth grade, but he works in a supermarket now. But people tell me that it is a waste that my son is not in school. He will have no future without education. But our situation is very bad. I really want to send him to school, but at the same time we are in deep need of financial help. (interview with Layla, Beirut, 2014)

In the Bekaa Valley, some press has reported that displaced Syrians with no savings have accepted very low wages to provide their families with food. This has raised hostility among local Lebanese who see the Syrian workers as a threat to their own livelihoods, resulting in increased social discrimination and vigilantism. Other villagers, with more sympathetic *mukhtars* (mayors), have organized Syrian laborers effectively and thus reduced local expressions of antipathy. One district official told a researcher visiting an informal tented settlement that they "had no refugees" in his locality, even though over two thousand Syrians there were registered with the UNHCR. What he meant was that most of the Syrians had previously been in the village as seasonal laborers, and now had returned to settle more permanently with their families following the beginning of the conflict in Syria. These laborers were taking on familiar work and were not regarded as threatening to local Lebanese livelihoods (Janmyr and Mourad 2018, 554.).

Some Lebanese landowners have charged Syrians exorbitant fees to pitch a tent or a tarpaulin haphazardly on agricultural fields or wasteland. Others have organized the Syrians and helped them to pitch tents following a grid system on the margins of their villages. An employee for the International Rescue Committee (IRC) described one arrangement:

> Because the Lebanese government didn't allow international organizations to interfere and do formal tented settlements like they did in other countries, the solution here, for example, [is] for a big landowner to ask a guy to set up tents and be responsible. This person becomes a *shawish*. . . . Organizations would talk to him to distribute assistance, so he would have much more power compared to other people. . . . And he would have the biggest tent, and toilets close to his tent, since he is the only one with direct contact with the organizations. (national IRC employee, Zahle, May 2015)

The traditional *shawish* are gang masters or middlemen who for decades have organized seasonal work for Lebanon's agricultural sector in the Bekaa Valley. These shawish have now become liaisons between displaced Syrians and the international humanitarian architecture. They have thus been imbued with significant power in making decisions regarding who receives humanitarian assistance and other services and have been implicated in cases of violence and corruption. Although among the displaced and aid practitioners there is a shared understanding of who is a "vulnerable" person, there is little transparency in who actually receives humanitarian assistance from the larger international agencies and how those decisions are made. One Syrian living in an informal settlement expressed frustration and confusion:

> I just do not understand why I was cut off [of assistance]. You are supposed to be a family of five, and we are five: my wife, my two children, and my mother. And there is no one else to provide for the family. My neighbors, they are still on [assistance], and they have two males who can work. (Syrian man, Bekaa Valley, 2017, quoted in Janmyr and Mourad 2018, 550)

Many Syrians, despite their long association with Lebanon over decades and often close kinship ties, feel frightened and cut off from Lebanese society. Access to public hospitals, which are of limited number, is not available to displaced Syrians, and education in Lebanon's government schools is difficult to obtain. Nearly 60 percent of school-age Syrian children are not receiving education (Chatty et al. 2014). Although some international NGOs and national and local NGOs operate in Beirut and in the Bekaa Valley to provide basic needs, there is little interaction with the Lebanese host community, except where local municipality leaders and grassroots organizations have taken matters into their own hands. In interviews, little evidence emerged of host community involvement in any "survival in dignity" activity on an individual basis; NGO activity was limited to more "distant and distancing" charity work or local civil society efforts in Beirut organized by middle-class Lebanese and Syrians resident in the country. The UNHCR's slow implementation of cash assistance to the most needy and vulnerable Syrians in Lebanon has resulted in large numbers of women and children being seen on the streets of Beirut begging—something generally scorned and regarded with little sympathy by the Lebanese and some international aid workers.

JORDAN

Syrians in Jordan have a more formally recognized relationship with a strong state structure. Jordanian officials claim there are over one million "displaced" Syrians in the country, creating a burden that the state demands be met by international humanitarian assistance. This is an overestimation, much as has been seen in earlier refugee crises (Marfleet and Chatty 2009). To clarify, the population of Jordan is about ten million; officially, some six hundred thousand Syrians are temporary guests in the country. Another six hundred thousand or so were already regular residents in the country. So only half the Syrians present in the country have arrived since the start of armed conflict in Syria in 2011. Whatever the numbers, Syrians regard Jordan's initial response to the humanitarian crisis—and to the mass influx of people from Syria's southern border towns, including Der'aa and adjacent tribal areas—as open and generous. Most of these Syrians had kinship ties in northern Jordan or well-established social networks, which helped the displaced Syrians to find local accommodation. So relatively few Syrians were forced into the refugee camps set up by the United Nations near the border with Syria.

There are three major camps in Jordan: The first to open and most important is Za'tari, which housed as many as 180,000 people in 2014 but is currently down to 80,000 residents. Initially the international aid architecture's policy in running the camps was to tightly control accommodation and food allocation. This resulted in demonstrations, disturbances, and general unrest in the camp until Syrians were allowed to set up their own shopping street and rearrange their accommodations to bring dignity to their social interactions. The humanitarian aid architecture took "lessons learned" from this experience to build a new camp, Azraq and—rather than model the new camp's design according to the Syrians' preferences—completely removed any agency from the Syrian refugees and significantly removed any self-expression or autonomous social life from the camp.

Over time, the Jordanian government has restricted access to the country and actively prevented some, such as unaccompanied male youth, from entering, or returned others, such as Palestinian refugees from Syria. One aid practitioner explained the shift:

> At the beginning you had a refugee crisis with a security component, and it has since become a security crisis with a refugee component. So, in the early days it was "these are our brothers," and so the natural generosity has now given way to more suspicion about who these people are, and the security card is played all the time now. (senior international practitioner, Amman, 2015)

The problem in Jordan is that Syrians are being treated as temporary guests—whereas in Lebanon, they were regarded as temporary workers. In Jordan, Syrians have no right to work. In fact, it is considered a criminal offense if they do. After their initial few months in the country, however, most Syrians realize that they must find work—generally in the informal economy—to support themselves and their families. If caught working, they are at risk of being deported to Syria or sent to one of the United Nations camps, Za'tari or Azraq. Yet the Syrians in Jordan prefer to work rather than seek charity assistance. One Syrian I spoke with told me:

> I am a carpenter. I have a skill. I do not want to go begging [to a charity]. If I can work to feed my family, that is better. I am ready to train Jordanians to be carpenters. That way I can be useful and give something back to this country. (Syrian carpenter from Der'aa, Amman, 2015)

Jordan has long been a country of asylum for refugees, starting with the mass influx of Palestinians after the 1947–1948 war over Palestine. Over the decades, it has constructed a set of procedures and institutions to actively encourage the involvement of the international humanitarian architecture. The country's exaggeration of refugee numbers was first noticed during the Iraqi refugee crisis of 2006–2007, when Jordan claimed to have received over a million Iraqis. The doubling of the number of Syrians in the current crisis is therefore not unexpected. And there is reason behind such calculations. Jordan has few natural resources other than potash, and tourism is an important part of its national income. So, too, are refugees. In some ways Jordan has become a refugee rentier state (Tsourapas 2019). Both international aid and bilateral assistance provide for infrastructural development in the country first, and refugee assistance second. This aid is manifested in the presence of a great many international organizations in Amman—so much so that several upper-middle-class sectors of the city have been transformed by a kind of humanitarian aid "tourism." The presence of these international organizations and NGOs is such that local NGOs and grassroots associations working directly with displaced Syrians are not nearly as prevalent as they are, for example, in Lebanon. This creates space for greater misunderstandings and confounding assumptions.

A discrepancy has emerged between what is widely written about Syrians in the local press—that Syrians are a burden on the Jordanian economy—and what policymakers and practitioners feel is occurring. Many policymakers believe that Syrians contribute more greatly to the Jordanian economy than is widely being written about and circulated in polite society. In an interview, one Jordanian policymaker emphasized that some World Bank reports were suggesting that the unemployment rate in Jordan initially had dropped by 2 percent since the start of the Syrian crisis due to "the surge in Syrian-owned factories opening [200] and the heavy employment of Jordanians [estimated at about 6,000]" (senior Jordanian economist, February 2015). This early investment in Jordan by Syrian businessmen—moving their factories from Syria to Jordan—is largely acknowledged but underplayed. The diversity across Syrians in terms of socioeconomic status, ethnicity, religion, culture, daily life, and social interaction, though understood at the local level, is more complex than policymakers seem to realize. Humanitarian aid practitioners and their reports fail to capture this diversity across locations in Jordan, referring to Syrians more generally in analyzing, for example, complex issues such as early marriage and gender-based violence (Rabo 2008; Stevens 2016; CARE International 2016, UNICEF 2013). In addition, with nearly 80 percent of displaced Syrians self-settled, house visits by NGOs to assess vulnerability and what further assistance might be made often become a spectacle of performance: Syrians host the humanitarian aid visitor and perform "refugee vulnerability and neediness" in order to receive assistance (Wagner 2018).

Thus, the host community in Jordan is bombarded with stereotypes and negative reporting regarding the influence of Syrian refugees in the country—although this reporting is not backed up by emerging studies. Curiously, at the same time, there is widespread acknowledgment that Syrians are skilled workmen, especially carpenters. Employment in the informal sector has created stress among Syrians, even though the work brings in much-needed funds. Syrians who work are continuously anxious and fearful of arrest, as they have no work permits—even though they are largely replacing Egyptians, not Jordanians, in the work force:

> Syrian refugees are skilled craftsmen, especially carpenters, we all know that. Jordanians are not skilled carpenters. Syrians are not taking jobs from Jordanians; but they may be taking jobs from Egyptians. They are working informally, but that puts a lot of stress on them because they can be arrested and deported if they are found out. (senior Jordanian policymaker, 2015)

Some social discrimination is leveled at Syrians in Jordan, but it is muted compared with that expressed in Lebanon. Even though the majority of Syrians in Irbid and Amman, Lebanon, are tied in "real" rather than fictive kinship, the negative social attitudes of Jordanians are kept closer to the chest. This may be due to tribal custom and general conceptual concerns related to the requirement of hospitality to tribal kin and others in patron/client relationships (many Syrians from the Der'aa region are associated with the Beni Khalid tribal confederation also found in northern Jordan). Jordanians generally do recognize that the country benefits—from international aid—from its expenditure on refugees, and that a significant percentage goes into government projects to assist Jordanians. The bilateral aid agreement announced between the United States and Jordan in 2015—in which the United States said it would increase assistance to Jordan to $1 billion per year over three years—was meant to address Jordan's "short-term, extraordinary needs," according to the US State Department, including its efforts to combat the Islamic State and assistance for refugees from Iraq and Syria. In practice, those funds first went to infrastructure development and the construction of fifty high schools for Jordanians—after which funds were spent to address the needs of refugees.

TURKEY

Turkey, hosting close to four million displaced Syrians, is the most interesting case among the three countries discussed here. Syrians in Turkey have flooded into areas that are most like their own, in the sense of shared identity and ethnic belonging, with areas along the modern southern border of Turkey seeing the heaviest concentration of the displaced. The city of Gaziantep is particularly noteworthy as a magnet for Syrian investment that has improved the economy of southern Turkey tremendously over the past two decades. Indeed, trade links between this part of Turkey and Aleppo go back to at least Ottoman times (see Figures 4.3 and 4.4).

Syrians in Turkey come from a variety of economic, religious, and ethnic backgrounds, as well as from various social classes. As one of my interlocutors told me:

> The upper and middle classes have largely found their way to urban centers like Istanbul, where they have rented property and set up businesses. They consider themselves immigrants, while most of those displaced Syrians who have crossed into Turkey but remained near the border regard themselves as refugees. (Syrian male researcher based in Istanbul, October 2014)

Many of the displaced Syrians I met in Turkey expressed deep concern with the negative stereotypes of "dirty" and "uncouth" Arabs, commonly articulated by middle-class Turks. Furthermore, other Syrians I interviewed in Istanbul said they were dismayed that so many Turkish observers had difficulty differentiating between the general Syrian refugee population and the *nawwar*—peripatetic, largely Romani Gypsy communities found in Turkey, as well as in Iraq and Syria. Many nawwar have been displaced by the Syrian crisis and are commonly seen begging on the streets of Istanbul,

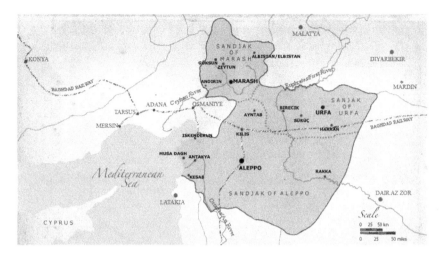

Figure 4.3. The province (vilayet) of Aleppo at the beginning of the 20th century. Map clearly demarcating the province of Aleppo up to World War One. The horizontal dotted line across what seems the middle of the province is the border established between the French- mandated Syria and the newly created Republic of Turkey, thus severing families, as well as business, social, and religious communities across an international frontier.

Source: www.houshamadyan.org.

Ankara, and other cities. Largely unrecognized, the Gypsies of southwest Asia also have seen their largely seasonal economy disrupted by the armed conflicts in Iraq and Syria, and have gravitated to Turkey, where they can survive in greater security.

One Syrian woman resident in Istanbul, interviewed in October 2015, articulated Syrians' general discomfort with being associated with the nawwar. "The Turkish people think that any woman sitting on a street corner breastfeeding her infant, while begging, is a Syrian," she said. "They don't realize she is a nawwar."

In addition, street begging was widely condemned by both host community members and Syrian refugees. "I don't like to give money to beggars because it just encourages them," one Turkish aid practitioner said in an interview in 2014. In an interview in 2015, a phone-shop owner who employed several Syrian youths said, "I do not like begging, and I will not give to beggars, but I do give to individual Syrians I know who are in need."

Unlike Jordan, Turkey did not accept assistance from the UNHCR in managing its Syrian refugee flow. Although the UNHCR first began working in Turkey in 1991—at Van, after the 1990 Gulf War—it has been permitted to advise the Turkish government in only four areas: registration, camp

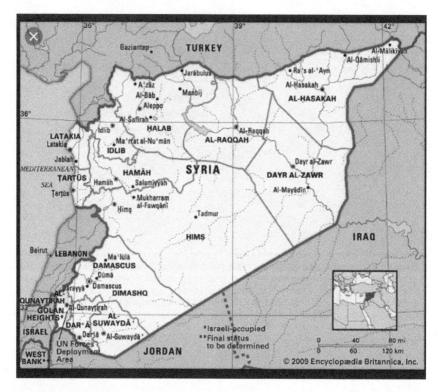

Figure 4.4. Map showing Syria's modern borders taking in about half of the previous province of Ottoman Aleppo.
Source: Encyclopedia Britannica.

management, civil society capacity in camps, and voluntary return (senior UNHCR official in Turkey, October 2015). Instead, AFAD, the Prime Minister Disaster and Emergency Management Presidency, undertook building the first twenty-five refugee camps for 250,000 displaced Syrians. The International Crisis Group (ICG) labeled these "the best refugee camps ever seen" (ICG 2014). I would perhaps identify them as "temporary towns" with a focus not only on food and shelter, but also health, security, social activities, education, communications, interpretation, banking, and vocational training. Moreover, their reliance on national and local, not international, staff to run the camps displayed a sensitivity to Syrians' desire for dignity and agency. The director of one camp told me, in an interview near Gaziantep in October 2015, that when the camp first opened, the Turkish government had provided three meals a day. "But the Syrian people did not like our food," he said. "And so the government decided to give them their own supermarkets and let them buy what they needed. It made the people happier, and it turned out to be a big savings for the Turkish government."

A sentiment of recognizing and acting on the needs of Syria's refugees was widely articulated by members of local Turkish host communities. The importance of this third sector—charitable organizations and religious-/Sufi-based associations—in providing assistance was pronounced, and many local associations were heavily supported by government and local donations. The largest of these organizations, IHH (Humanitarian Relief Foundation), works in over one hundred countries and provides relief in cases of war, earthquakes, hunger, and conflict. Although it is funded almost entirely by contributions from Turkey's merchant religious class, it is closely associated with the prime minister's political agenda and is sometimes referred to as a governmental nongovernment organization. Nevertheless, it has played a large role in providing humanitarian assistance to displaced Syrians in the absence of many international organizations that have been unable to secure permits to operate in the country, or that have been shut down after years of successful operations (e.g., Mercy Corps as reported in *The New York Times*, March 2017).

Widespread support from civil society was especially noticeable among established NGOs and religious organizations related to the Islamic Sufi sector of society (civil society rather than religious organizations). It was common in Istanbul and Gaziantep for neighborhood public kitchens providing free meals and bread to the poor to also provide sustenance to refugees resident in the area. One Syrian woman recounted her experience:

> My husband came first and then I joined him eight months later with our baby. At first, we went to Mersin, but my husband could not find a job. When we ran out of money we came to Gaziantep, because the Syrian Interim Government was here. We figured there would be more jobs here. So, we came here and two months later we met this nice man who found a job for my husband and rented us these two rooms. Our neighbors gave us some mattress and a TV to watch Syrian television. There is also a mosque nearby where I go and the people there give me diapers for the baby, bread, and daily hot meals, as well as supplies of sugar, pasta, and oil. (interview with Hala, Gaziantep, 2014)

In the first few years of the Syrian crisis, lack of communication from the government and a poor understanding of Syrians' situation led to demonstrations, arrests, and in the autumn of 2014 in Gaziantep and other cities to a dozen or so deaths. Many Turkish citizens felt that more transparency on the part of the government in terms of what Syrians were entitled to would have relieved the critical situation and growing discriminatory attitudes. Many thought that refugees from Syria were being given salaries by the Turkish government; others believed that Syrians were working for lower wages (their Turkish employers did not have to pay taxes), and that this was driving out unskilled Turkish workers who had no safety net when they lost their jobs to Syrians.

A lack of common language might have caused a divide in Turkey in other times, but in the current crisis, language seems to play a less significant role. In Lebanon and Jordan, speaking the same language has not helped educated Syrians to find work, as work was, and still is, prohibited for most categories of professional and skilled labor. In Turkey, however, professionals and skilled workers, unable to work in their métier during the early years of the crisis, were gradually allowed to do so. For example, after 2014, the Turkish government agreed to grant accreditation to any Syrian doctors who had trained outside Syria, especially if they agreed to work in the southern Turkish provinces, where more than 50 percent of displaced Syrians resided. Over all, in Turkey, being a "stranger" and speaking a different language seems to have encouraged greater sympathy and general support at the local community level.

THE IMPORTANCE OF HISTORY AND CONTEXT

Across the board, what emerges from research in Syria's neighboring countries is that history and social context matter. Many of the discrepancies between displaced Syrians, host community members and aid practitioners described above can be linked to historical social and kinship ties, as well as to political relations between Syria and Turkey, Syria and Lebanon, and Syria and Jordan. Disparity in perceptions among policymakers, aid practitioners, and host communities is widespread, but not equally so in the three countries.

In Lebanon, the consociational shape of governance and the long period during this crisis in which there was in effect no government led to a period of paralysis within the United Nations humanitarian aid system. During this period, the UN was unable to persuade Lebanon to permit it to establish formal refugee camps. Even the registration of refugees at the UNHCR was stopped at government request in 2015. Thus, effective relief programs such as cash transfer, meant to help the poorest and most vulnerable of Syrians, were late in getting started, resulting in an exponential rise in street begging and other "negative coping" strategies (pulling older children out of school to work; moving into structures unfit for human habitation; relying on former agricultural "gang masters" to act as liaisons with the UN humanitarian relief system). All these factors resulted in significant social discrimination and an unwillingness or inability among locals to help Syrians with basic health and education needs, though this was sometimes mitigated by the close ties and extended family networks among the very poor across the two countries. The lack of educational opportunity for nearly 60 percent of Syrian refugee children in Lebanon weighs heavily on the consciousness of their families. And a recent demand for "voluntary return" of Syrians to their country—especially among the March 8 Alliance politicians—is concerning.

In Jordan, the majority of Syrian refugees are closely linked to the Jordanian population, especially in northern Jordan, where close tribal ties are pronounced, and where original refuge was granted with host families related by blood or by marriage, particularly those fleeing from Der'aa and its surrounding villages. Jordanian sensitivity to the presence of Palestinian refugees from Syria (PRS) has resulted in draconian surveillance to identify such refugees, a dragnet that often pulls in non-Palestinian refugees from Syria. Those found to be illegally working are then deported across the border (if PRS) or to the Azraq or Za'tari camps, creating greater mistrust and suspicion of the host government by refugees from Syria. Educational opportunities are limited, and many Syrian children are able to attend only second-shift schools with inferior curriculum and reduced hours. Some Syrians consider the situation in Jordan so dire that they are preparing to return to Syria rather than face what they consider "inhuman conditions" any longer. As early as September 2015, UNHCR senior humanitarian aid practitioners in Jordan reported that two hundred Syrians were returning to Syria each day. These Syrians have continued to return not so much because they feel that doing so is safe—they are aware of the challenges of returning to a country that is neither safe nor at peace—but rather because their aspirations for living in safety and dignity in Jordan have gone unmet.

In Turkey, lessons learned have been more widely implemented in response to various critical events early in the Syrian crisis (e.g., demonstrations in October 2014) and to widespread criticism of the government's lack of transparency. The camps set up starting in 2012 by the Turkish emergency relief organization (AFAD)—without the assistance of UN experts and their camp templates—have rightly been described as having a "5-star rating" in terms of quality. These settlements were open, in that refugees could enter and leave daily. But absences of more than three weeks at a time were not tolerated, as a long list of Syrian exiles were waiting to gain access to the camps. As of 2019, many of these camps had been closed, and Turkish authorities had pushed Syrians into self-settlement and greater self-sufficiency in towns and villages. Furthermore, in 2019 Turkey held a second round of talks with the UNHCR, in an effort to work collaboratively on the safe and dignified voluntary return of Syrians to their country—this before any measures could be taken to guarantee safe return to a country still fighting rebels in the Idlib province (UNHCR 2019). It has been estimated that some 200,000 to 250,000 Syrians have been "refouled" to Syria, mainly men who have been found residing outside the regions of Turkey where they first registered as displaced.

Although interviews in Turkey took place in January 2015, before the announcement of domestic law providing Syrians with formal IDs and temporary protection (including rights to health and education opportunities and permission to apply for work permits), it was clear even then that Turkey was far more humane and practical in its approach to the mass influx of refugees from Syria than were Lebanon and Jordan—despite a language barrier that did not exist in Lebanon or Jordan. Turkey had the least public expression of social discrimination, and Sufi-based organizations were actively providing assistance at the local community level—mainly hot meals and community-supported accommodation. Many members of such organizations expressed their concern about providing refuge to Syrians, out of religious and ethical obligations. In addition, social cohesion in Turkey has been strong, which bodes well for Syrians' eventual local integration in Turkey, or for their return to Syria as a "friendly and supportive neighboring state," depending on which political solution finally emerges. Even Turkey's announcement on February 27, 2020 that it would open its borders to Europe did not result in a stream of Syrians crossing; most of the ten thousand people who attempted to reach Europe in that wave were from Afghanistan, Iran, and Iraq (Amnesty International 2020).

TOWARD A COMPREHENSIVE PLAN OF ACTION

It is ironic that Turkey, the one country that has not requested assistance from the UNHCR, seems to have managed the process of providing assistance to the displaced without undermining refugee agency and dignity. Largely working alone with local Turkish staff drawn from the Turkish civil service—as well as staff from AFAD and IHH, the main quasi-official Turkish NGO—Turkey has managed the Syrian refugee crisis with relative sensitivity and concern. The separate histories of Turkey, Lebanon, and Jordan have obviously contributed to the disparities in perceptions, aspirations, and behavior among refugees, host community members, and aid practitioners in each of the three countries. The moderated engagement of the international humanitarian aid architecture in Turkey—compared with its greater engagement in Lebanon and Jordan—has also contributed to some of the disparities noted in this study.

Global templates for humanitarian assistance built from experiences in very different contexts and among populations of significantly different makeup are not easily integrated into Middle Eastern concepts of refuge, hospitality, and charity. The close social ties and networks of Syrians in Lebanon and Jordan, but not in Turkey, have meant that the initial generosity among relatives in a wide social network has more rapidly given way to hostility and discrimination. This differs with the situation in Turkey, where fewer Syrians had close kinship networks (with the exception of those in the Hatay province—formerly Syrian Alexandretta—which was ceded to Turkey in 1939 during the French Mandate), and where original hosting arrangements were based on a religious and ethical sense of duty to the stranger.

The disparity in perceptions among refugees, members of local hosting communities, and aid practitioners is especially pronounced in Lebanon and Jordan, where the international humanitarian aid architecture is the most active. The use of UN frameworks in creating an architecture of assistance is built upon templates developed over the past few decades largely among agrarian and poor developing countries. Such policy and practice do not fit easily into the middle-income countries of the Eastern Mediterranean, among a refugee population that is largely educated and middle-class. Without a serious effort to make humanitarian "solutions" fit the context of the Middle East, success will continue to be muted, at best, and damaging, at worst.

Many refugees and aid practitioners articulated steps the Western aid agencies, the United Nations, and the European Union could take to ameliorate conditions, reduce the dangerous journeys via smugglers across the Mediterranean, and create conditions on the ground for future return and reintegration in Syria. It was clear from all interviews with displaced Syrians that self-settlement was preferred to encampment. The former was seen as creating better conditions for local accommodation and potentially a return and reintegration into Syria's many social communities. (Lessons learned from Bosnia Herzegovina support this position [Blitz 2015].) Self-settlement helped give displaced Syrians agency to work with local hosting communities and the international aid architecture to create programs and projects drawing on their own professional skills. This, in turn, allowed for the creation of local community drop-in centers offering opportunities for informal education and technical training, for Syrians and local residents alike. Skills development, psychosocial support, and language instruction were regularly suggested as measures to assist in local accommodation, and to pave the way for a better future for the current lost generation of Syrian youth, as well as for youth in the host country. Lessons learned from the UNHCR's drop-in centers established in Syria for Iraqi refugees were referred to as exemplary. With the exception of Turkey, which was quick to organize Temporary Education Centers (teaching in Arabic), there have been scarce opportunities for Syria's displaced youth to continue their education in other countries, despite numerous studies pointing to education gaps and opportunities. This has rendered the UN slogan, "No Lost Generation," no more than that—a slogan.

Temporary protection, not resettlement, is the main aspiration for those who have been forced to flee Syria to work and educate their youth, until such time as they can return to their country. The temporary protection afforded to nearly 1.2 million Bosnians during the 1992–1995 war in Europe is a good example of what the European states might do again if they have the will.

The current situation is unsustainable. Lebanon and Jordan, and even Turkey, cannot accommodate the vast numbers of displaced Syrians flowing into their countries for much longer. Throwing money and favorable international financing via various EU institutions to regional hosting states also cannot go on much longer. Without a dramatic change in policy and programming, Syrians will continue to resort to flight from the region by any means necessary, to secure survival in dignity—an opportunity to work to feed and educate their families until they can return to Syria—which they thus far have been unable to widely access. The current focus on voluntary return to Syria cannot be regarded as the one durable solution. Instead, the humanitarian aid architecture must consider earlier successful solutions, such as the Comprehensive Plan of Action for Indochinese Refugees, initiated for the Vietnamese and Laotian "boat people" in 1989 (Casella 2016). In that case, after years of negotiations, the UNHCR succeeded in dramatically expanding the screening of asylum seekers for refugee status. Those denied such status were repatriated/returned to Vietnam, but only after the state had agreed not to impose penalties for "illegal departure," which was monitored by the UNHCR. Others, who had self-settled and were living in safety and dignity, were allowed to remain in their host countries. Only a comprehensive plan of action—one that includes the aspirations and concerns of displaced Syrians, their host states, and their country of origin, as well as the backing and support of the UNHCR and Europe—can offer a solution to the population movement that has emerged from the Syrian humanitarian crisis.

REFERENCES

Amnesty International. 2020. "Caught in a Political Game: Asylum-Seekers and Migrants on the Greek/Turkey Border Pay the Price for Europe's Failures." https://www.amnesty.org/download/Documents/EUR0120772020ENGLISH. PDF.

Blitz, B. 2015. "Bosnia Revisited: A Retrospective on the Legacy of Conflict." *Forced Migration Review* 50: 49–51.

CARE International. 2016. "On Her Own: How Women Forced to Flee from Syria Are Shouldering Increased Responsibility as They Struggle to Survive." https://www.care-international.org/files/files/CARE_On-Her-Own_refugee-media-report_Sept-2016.pdf.

Casella, Alexander. 2016. "Managing the 'Boat People' Crisis: The Comprehensive Plan of Action for Indochinese Refugees." *Desperate Migration Series No. 2.* International Peace Institute.

Chatty, Dawn. 2010. *Displacement and Dispossession in the Modern Middle East.* Cambridge: Cambridge University Press.

Chatty, Dawn. 2014. "Anthropology and Forced Migration." In *The Oxford Handbook of Refugee and Forced Migration Studies*, edited by Elene Fiddian-Qasmiyeh, Gil Loescher, Katy Long, and Nando Sigona, pp. 74–75. Oxford: Oxford University Press.

Chatty, Dawn, Hashem Ahmadzadeh, Metin Çorabatır, Leen Hashem, Jalal Al Husseini and Sarah Wahby. 2014. "Ensuring Quality Education for Young Refugees from Syria (12–25 Years)." Refugee Studies Centre, Oxford Department of International Development, University of Oxford. http://www.rsc.ox.ac.uk/files/publications/other/rr-syria-youth-education-2014.pdf.

Chatty, Dawn. 2017. "How Syrian Refugees Survive." *Current History: A Journal of Contemporary World Affairs* 116 (794): 337–342.

Gladstone, Rick. 2017. "Turkey Halts Mercy Corps, Charity That Aids Over 500,000 Syrians a Month. *New York Times*, March 8.

International Crisis Group. 2014. "Blurring the Borders: Syria Spillover Risks for Turkey." Europe Report #225. 30 April, Brussels.

Janmyr, Maja, and Lama Mourad. 2018. "Modes of Ordering: Labelling, Classification, and Categorization in Lebanon's Refugee Response. *Journal of Refugee Studies* 31 (4): 544–565.

Krulfeld, Ruth M., and Jeffery L. Macdonald, Eds. 1998. *Power, Ethics, and Human Rights: Anthropological Studies of Refugee Research and Action.* Boston and Oxford: Rowman & Littlefield.

Marfleet, Philip, and Dawn Chatty. 2009. "Iraq's Refugees—Beyond Tolerance." Forced Migration Policy Briefing 4. Refugee Studies Centre, University of Oxford.

Rabo, Annika. 2008. "'Doing Family': Two Cases in Contemporary Syria." *Hawwa* 6 (2):129–153.

Stevens, Matthew R. 2016. "The Collapse of Social Networks Among Syrian Refugees in Urban Jordan." *Contemporary Levant* 1 (1): 51–63.

Tsourapas, Gerasimos. 2019. "The Syrian Refugee Crisis and Foreign Policy Decision-Making in Jordan, Lebanon, and Turkey." *Journal of Global Security Studies* 4 (4): 464–481.

Wagner, Ann-Christin. 2018. "Giving Aid Inside the Home: Humanitarian House Visits, Performative Refugeehood, and Social Control of Syrians in Jordan." *Migration and Society: Advances in Research* 1 (1): 36–50.

UNHCR. 2019. "UNHCR and Turkey Hold Further Discussions on Voluntary Repatriation of Syrian Refugees." November 29. https://www.unhcr.org/uk/news/press/2019/11/5de123694.html.

UNHCR. 2020. "UNHCR Statement on the Situation at the Turkey–EU Border." March 2. https://www.unhcr.org/uk/news/press/2020/3/5e5d08ad4/unhcr-statement-situation-turkey-eu-border.html.

UNICEF. 2013. "Shattered Lives: Challenges and Priorities for Syrian Children and Women in Jordan." June 10. https://www.unicef.org/infobycountry/files/Shattered_Lives_June10.pdf.

CHAPTER 5

The Business of Conflict

Humanitarian Assistance and the War Economy in Syria

DUNCAN MCLEAN

A striking and darkly amusing comparison was made in the early years of Médecins Sans Frontières's (MSF) medical support to besieged populations in Syria. To provide some perspective, it was noted that the cost of one day's aerial bombardment would be equivalent to seventy-eight hundred MSF donations, meaning "MSF could bomb for less than two hours"; one day of fighting to hold or take a government position would require seven to fourteen donations; and the cost of "one anti-tank missile" in a besieged area would roughly equal a single donation, or about $10,000. Keeping in mind that each MSF-supported location "will get at best and in the most critical situation eight donations a year" we can be collectively reassured (MSF, internal document, "Comparison Between Medical Donation & Weapon Cost," undated).

Of course, the authors knew it is almost impossible to determine what happens to lost cash, and the comparison is somewhat disingenuous given that "remote-controlled bombs, for example, can be built for a few hundred dollars" (Shanahan 2018). But the sense of proportion is intriguing. And the description of caricatured eye-catching diversions provides a useful reminder that it is not the extreme cases that represent the greatest risk. Much like the "extensive international focus on financing prohibited parties," both fail to recognize the "true threat of humanitarian aid

Duncan McLean, *The Business of Conflict* In: *Everybody's War.* Edited by: Jehan Bseiso, Michiel Hofman, and Jonathan Whittall, Oxford University Press. © Médecins Sans Frontières 2021. DOI: 10.1093/oso/9780197514641.003.0006 diversion: a systematic and pervasive war economy" (Humanitarian Access Team, Mercy Corps, pers. comm., March 2018).

Although humanitarian assistance inevitably plays a role in the political economy of any given conflict, arguably it has been taken to a new level in Syria (Carbonnier 2015, 68).[1] Over the course of nine years of fighting, a vast and deeply entrenched war economy has developed to encompass multiple transactions, both financial and commodity-based. Profits have been dispersed to all sides, further complicated by the clear financial interest of some in pursuing hostilities irrespective of their political or ideological leanings. Western sanctions, intended to pressure the Syrian government into moderating its behavior, have reinforced the entire system by actively encouraging an underground economy, all the while strengthening the authorities at the expense of the population.

This chapter will analyze the evolution of Syria's war economy and the role unwittingly played by humanitarian assistance, including medical support provided by MSF. Formally besieged areas such as East Ghouta will be examined in detail, raising a number of troubling questions as to the limits humanitarian organizations are prepared to accept when operating in a broader system of corruption, predation, and denial of access.

PRE-UPRISING ANTECEDENTS

The Syrian war economy has been described as "a vast ecosystem of illicit profiteering, where the worst of enemies are also partners in business" (Lund 2018). Understanding this state of affairs requires looking back at the profound economic changes that were taking place in the decade preceding the 2011 uprising. Economic liberalization had led to the privatization of most public services, including "various vegetable, fruit, and meat companies, textile companies, the postal service, telecommunications, public construction, transportation, and banking services" (Humanitarian Access Team, Mercy Corps, pers. comm., March 2018).[2]

These policies resulted in two simultaneous trends: They gave elites opportunities for significant wealth accumulation while "increasing their dependence on the state." More important, those who most benefited had close ties to the presidential administration, including family members, close associates, and influential supporters. Meanwhile most small businesses "remained on the peripheries of economic gains and political power" (Abboud 2017). Put more bluntly, business leaders needed access to the political elite to exploit the new economic policies, and the government needed those same businesses to generate growth and revenue (Abboud 2013).

A second essential aspect to consider when reviewing the pre-uprising economic situation is the historic levels of corruption. Doing business in Syria has been described by one observer as "never a good way to keep your hands clean," with the periods of Presidents Hafez al-Assad and his son Bashar gaining a "well-deserved reputation not only for authoritarianism, but also for graft and greed" (Lund 2018). This is certainly borne out in corruption analyses. According to Transparency International, Syria already was ranked 127 worldwide on its Corruption Perceptions Index in 2010 and since has descended to 178th place out of 180 countries.[3]

In other words, the war did not make the war economy alone; the seeds were already there. And the "same veins of corruption that existed before the war exist now; many have simply taken advantage of the situation" (MSF staff, interview, Berlin, March 22, 2018). Indeed it has been argued that there is a clear element of continuity in the "inequality and racketeering" seen in Syria prior to 2011 and today: "If anything, the conflict seems to have left the Syrian business elite even more crooked and conceited, and ordinary people even more exploited and despondent." Combined with the growth of diverse opposition groups and their own commercial interests, business interests now compete "more openly and more violently than in the pre-2011 era, when transactions took place under the umbrella of the police state" (Lund 2018).

THE ECONOMICS OF STATE SURVIVAL

Highlighting the underlying aspects of Syria's economic decline is not to disregard the central element of the conflict itself, wherein "nearly all economic activity is necessarily connected in some way to the war economy and stakeholders within the Syrian government" (Humanitarian Access Team, Mercy Corps, pers. comm., March 2018). Irrespective of liberalization policies and preexisting levels of corruption, the war also has accelerated the creation of a "new class of elites" who owe their fortunes to the conflict and are "implicated in violence even when they do not directly perpetuate it" (Abboud 2017). And as importantly, warlords have emerged on all sides who "benefit personally from the status quo and provide important sources of funding to their backers." Arguably almost "every detail in the war is being squeezed for profit" (Sinjab 2017).

This shift did not occur overnight but rather evolved during the first few years of the conflict. Certainly, consumption and investment dropped rapidly with the disappearance of tourism and the "broad loss of domestic confidence." Foreign currency reserves were hit in the first phase of Western sanctions, notably oil revenue, of which 90 percent was exported to the European Union. By the conflict's second year, the manufacturing base had collapsed, given that roughly half of major factories were based in and around Damascus and Aleppo. The expansion of violence particularly in Aleppo "was part of a broader breakdown in law and order and growing reports of kidnappings and lootings." Finally, the government loss of the northeast in the spring of 2013, the base of most oil and grain resources, further increased "dependence on international backers for oil and credit facilities" (Yazigi 2014).

Consequently, by 2014, extreme economic contraction was evident. In brute impersonal terms, the budget deficit had accelerated exponentially, government revenues had declined drastically, and inflation was at 30 percent (World Bank 2016). Economic activity indicated a "rapid decline in every sector, with total economic activity contracting more than 60 percent from its level before the conflict" (Abboud 2017). The dire economic straits of the Syrian government at the time raises questions as to how it survived, particularly as "most areas under regime control" continued to have access to basic state amenities such as "water, electricity, education, and health services, and commodities such as bread, fruit and vegetables, gasoline, and heating oil" (Yazigi 2014).

Described as the "financial resilience of the regime," several key factors came into play in the government's attempt to ensure the support of its core constituency. Although basic services were maintained, there was a severe reduction in domestic expenditures including fuel subsidies and infrastructure spending. There was also a clampdown on businesses to ensure a minimal tax revenue along with increased custom tariffs that contributed to a fall in domestic demand (Jihad Yazigi, interview, March 22, 2018; Yazigi 2014). Even the much-vaunted payment of civil servants irrespective of location was erratic, unchanged since 2011 despite inflation, and "only paid when it suited the regime" (Dr. Reinoud Leenders, interview, King's College London, April 12, 2018; Tokmajyan 2016).

External aspects of government resilience included a shift in support, notably a dramatic increase from Iran and Russia as traditional trading partners such as Turkey and Saudi Arabia aligned themselves with opposition groups. Iran provided credit lines totaling "somewhere between $4.5 and $6 billion," one for petrol and at least one more for imports and services supplied by Iranian entities. Russia meanwhile facilitated access to several of its banks for Syrian assets previously held in European financial institutions but subject to sanctions (Jihad Yazigi, interview, March 22, 2018; Yazigi 2014).[4]

Although a measure of central authority continued to exist in government-controlled areas, it was by no means complete, as demonstrated by the reliance on armed militias. Provided a degree of "local leverage and autonomy," the pillaging of areas retaken from the opposition has been especially common (Yazigi 2014). The conversion of Shabiha militiamen to "popular committees," then "National Defense Forces," and finally warlords is a case in point. Their rapid accumulation of wealth was a result of having been given "the green light by the regime to earn whatever they can get however they can get it in return for loyalty" (Sinjab 2017).

Neither have the myriad opposition groups been starved of resources, despite the reverse phenomenon of state collapse in areas under their control. By 2015, unemployment in opposition areas was estimated to range between 60 and 90 percent, "making people vulnerable to combat recruitment," the only growth industry beyond the humanitarian sector (Turkmani et al. 2015). And with the collapse of security, an "informal economy comprising looting, kidnapping, and smuggling" became a significant source of income (Yazigi 2014).

Another important source of income for opposition groups and government-aligned forces can be found at border crossings and checkpoints, along with related smuggling operations—a situation where allegiances became negotiable (Sherlock 2013).[5] Meanwhile, the northeastern region "developed an economic life of its own" as smugglers refined oil themselves, after which it was "exported to Turkey or resold to other parts of the country." It has been argued that the expansion of the war economy in these areas has been "particularly fueled by the intra-rebel fight for lucrative resources such as border posts, oil fields, and grain storehouses" (Yazigi 2014). Certainly for some, the funding of military actions remained an objective, although others had clearly "given up the fight against the regime to run operations that line their own pockets" (Sherlock 2013).

As idealism gave way to cynicism in the years after the initial uprising, it was already becoming evident to some observers that "significant sectors of the economy" were thriving off the conflict. More disturbingly, as the war economy came to replace and dominate economic life, it was "creating incentives for those now making money from the conflict to prolong it" (Yazigi 2014). And as President Assad's "untouchable caste of regime-linked private-sector tycoons" grew in wealth and influence, corruption "mutated into a many-headed hydra of armed actors running their own rent-seeking operations and trade networks." This has provided fertile ground for the emergence of an army of brokers, fixers, and conflict traders (Lund 2018). For those middlemen, along with individuals and groups "on both sides of the divide," the conflict has cemented "lucrative new money-making opportunities" (Yazigi 2014).

An obvious example can be seen in basic procurement. With prices "inflated due to access restrictions imposed by parties to the conflict," monopolies over specific commodities were purchased by local businessmen from "those same political and military elites who imposed and maintain access restrictions." In other words, suffering was "monetized by those responsible for its occurrence in the first place" (Humanitarian Access Team, Mercy Corps, pers. comm., March 2018).

Speculation over the weakened Syrian pound also offered new opportunities by allowing those close to the presidential administration to capitalize on the "differential between the official and black-market rates" in order to make large profits (Yazigi 2014). Money laundering added further pressure on the Syrian pound. Multiple networks were developed to this end: Hawala, front companies, banking services in friendly countries— "much of this visibly facilitating high-end real estate construction outside Damascus" (international donor, interview, March 16, 2018).

So even as Syria's "rebels, Kurdish nationalists, and Assad loyalists fight and kill each other," they also trade and, in some cases, grow rich. Meanwhile middlemen and brokers "provide the connective tissue" of conflict services connecting the front lines (Lund 2018). They ensure completion of "transactions and payments that maintain the flow of goods and materials into regime areas, while businesspeople in the Turkish borderlands secure the flow of goods to rebel groups" (Abboud 2017). It's a situation depressingly described as market forces "doing their thing in a business environment regulated by military power rather than by laws and bureaucracies" (Lund 2018).

SELF-DEFEATING SANCTIONS

A final essential point before moving on to the humanitarian sector is the purported role and impact of sanctions. The war economy described, and the related opportunity to profit from the sieges, is not simply the result of historical antecedents, military strategy, or a rapacious business elite, but rather of a broader economic breakdown. The causes are numerous and include damage to infrastructure, along with the loss of oil and gas revenue. Printing money and emptying foreign reserves have hardly compensated

(*Economist* 2017). However, a constant since the beginning of the conflict, and one of the determining factors in how the entire Syrian war economy has evolved, has been the partial imposition of sanctions.

To begin with, it should be noted that sanctions are not under the auspices of the United Nations but rather are Western, consequently "many countries continue to trade with the Syrian regime" (Jihad Yazigi, interview, March 22, 2018). Nevertheless they are both "deep and far-reaching," eventually coming to include "a total arms embargo, restrictions on all imports of Syrian oil, bans on all forms of public and private financial support to Syria, bans of telecommunications equipment exports to Syria, prohibitions of financial transactions with Syrian financial institutions, and the control of exports to Syria of any goods or material that might be used for internal repression" (Abboud 2017).

It can credibly be argued, however, that as an unintended consequence, sanctions have directly benefitted the war economy. With state entities and officials tied to the presidential administration targeted, the Syrian authorities have sought "intermediaries for their international transactions, giving new individuals the opportunity to enrich themselves" (Yazigi 2014). And much like the middlemen and fixers facilitating trade across front lines, others have "helped the regime skirt sanctions, establishing front companies that import fuel, food and luxury items" (*Economist* 2017). Given the long history of sanctions and smuggling in the region, the shift to "new supply networks" is not difficult to imagine (Beechwood International 2015). The direct result has been personal enrichment for the few and the increasing price of basic goods for the many.

Even items not under sanction, such as food imports and medicine, have provided the opportunity for profit given the significant mark-up, incidentally influencing the expenses of humanitarian support (Saul 2013).[6] And on the reverse side, sanctions have given the presidential administration a convenient "scapegoat for the public cost" of the conflict, and increased dependence on its allies. In other words, Western-backed sanctions intended to "coerce the regime into accepting the demands of its population" have clearly failed, and, in fact, have reinforced the authorities (Yazigi 2014).

AID CHANNELED THROUGH DAMASCUS

As a starting point, humanitarian aid has been, at least partially, a "default foreign-policy instrument" in the Syrian context. Periodic public pressure from donor states to stop war crimes and crimes against humanity have been given the sop of humanitarian assistance in the place of any collective will to address either the root causes or extreme violence (Carbonnier 2015, 50). And much as with counterproductive sanctions, if aid is "used to relieve political pressure for lack of policy" (interview with MSF staff, Berlin, March 22, 2018) it would be a depressing irony if it also has played a role in perpetuating the Syrian conflict, or at least complicating a resolution. The obvious paradox needs to be underlined: The major supporters of sanctions—the European Union, the United States, and the United Kingdom—are simultaneously the "biggest funders of the humanitarian response that has undermined those sanctions" (Sparrow 2018).

This is neither to ignore the positive impact of humanitarian assistance nor to underestimate the extreme challenges aid organizations face. Physical insecurity for aid actors has been a constant since the beginning of the conflict, with organizations forced to work under "two or more rival regimes" while "negotiating a path among militant actors who routinely prey" on relief operations (Lund 2018). But given the risks of misused aid, an additional challenge exists as concerns the war economy.

Government-sanctioned aid represents by far the largest humanitarian input into Syria, unsurprisingly heavily biased toward areas under the control of the presidential administration. This has been by design, with a "well-established network of regime supporters that monopolize aid through the Ministry of Foreign Affairs to the Ministry of Defense all the way down to checkpoints" (international donor, interview with author and MSF staff, May 2018).[7] It is impossible to verify claims that "50 to 60 percent of all aid is skimmed from the regime," but it reasonably can be argued that to some degree "humanitarianism has been complicit" in the government's attempts to maintain power at any cost (Leenders and Mansour 2018, 225–57).

Given that the UN budget for Syria amounted to $5.2 billion between 2012 and 2016, it has received the brunt of such criticism, including accusations of unwittingly "throwing a lifeline to the regime that has no qualms about burning the entire country just to stay in power." Over the summer of 2016, specific critiques were being leveled at UN agencies over procurement practices and needs analysis. This included the agencies' use of local suppliers and individuals close to the presidential administration, and their "routinely" understating the number of "areas and people besieged by regime forces." An additional point of contention was the staffing of UN agencies in Damascus with "former Syrian ministry officials sympathetic to the regime" (Leenders 2016).

In their own defense, UN officials noted that the organization "can only work with a small number of partners approved by President Assad and that it does all it can to ensure the money is spent properly"

(Hopkins and Beals 2016b). In practice, the Syrian government has a list of "approved international and Syrian organizations and the UN cannot stray outside it" (Hopkins and Beals 2016a). The Syrian Arab Red Crescent (SARC) notably acts as the "gatekeeper" and "pivot" for UN humanitarian operations, and as the "main implementing partner for UN agencies," channeling roughly 60 percent of budgeted relief (Leenders and Mansour 2018, 225–57).

A breakdown of the 2015 UN response plan is revealing and provides substance to the critiques. Nine hundred million dollars of the plan's $1.1 billion budget was "funneled through Damascus, all of which is controlled to some extent by the Syrian authorities." This could include direct contributions such as blood bags donated by the WHO but managed by the Syrian Department of Defense, $5 million since the beginning of the conflict; or $11 million from the UN's Food and Agriculture Organization for operations run through the Ministry of Agriculture. Multiple businesses have been awarded local procurement contracts, with $4 million paid for fuel alone (Hopkins and Beals 2016a).

Support to charities close to the presidential administration also was favored and served political objectives. Syria Trust for Development, headed by First Lady Asma al-Assad and the al-Bustan Association, "tightly linked to senior regime incumbents," is the delivery partner of UNICEF and the International Organization for Migration. In these instances, sanctions are irrelevant, because despite their applying to individuals as well as state entities, the UN does not need to abide by partial Western-backed versions. Sanctions in this case again had the reverse effect, forcing UN agencies to rely on "large cash transfers" given the inaccessibility of the banking sector (Leenders and Mansour 2018, 225–57).

Justifications for such degrees of complicity should be familiar to most humanitarians. It is far from a perfect world, and shady compromises are a necessary part of humanitarian operations. A UN spokesman said as much when discussing the difficult choices made in Syria: "Faced with having to decide whether to procure goods or services from businesses that may be affiliated with the government or let civilians go without life-saving assistance, the choice is clear: our duty is to the civilians in need" (Hopkins and Beals 2016b). The United Nations Office for the Coordination of Humanitarian Affairs (OCHA) was more succinct and brutally honest in its own internal review, concluding that UN agencies "were simply not willing to jeopardize their operations in Syria by taking a tougher stance with the government."[8]

The negative publicity over the Syrian government's "manipulation of the relief effort" came to a head with the intensification of siege warfare in 2016, including reports that the authorities had "been allowed to edit the UN's aid plan." Another internal review followed with the modest recommendations of a workshop to "thrash out differences" and an ombudsman "to deal with complaints and ethical dilemmas for at least a year" (Beals 2018). Basic measures were not undertaken and despite the brief focus, little changed.

In the final tally, it can be argued that "aid might not keep the regime afloat, but it is significant," especially when UN procurement contracts "enter into the billions, parts of which go directly to the regime" (Dr. Reinoud Leenders, interview, King's College London, April 12, 2018). Clearly the decision to operate through Damascus not only reduced the impact of humanitarian assistance, it also "enabled the Assad regime to repurpose international funds for its own ends" (Sparrow 2018). It is also important to note that the siphoning of these resources did not occur instantaneously, nor through a series of dramatic events. Rather it has been systemic over a period of years, done with the active cooperation of UN humanitarian agencies, irrespective of the impact on the war economy or the war itself.

AID TO OPPOSITION-CONTROLLED AREAS

United Nation agencies have been criticized not only for "helping prop up a regime" but also for prioritizing "government-held areas" (Hopkins and Beals 2016b). They are certainly not alone in this regard, and it goes without saying that it is extremely difficult to undertake independent assessments and response in Syria, as demonstrated by Mercy Corps's being "forced to close its operations in Damascus because Syrian officials said it could not work in opposition-held areas of the country" (Chulov and Beals 2014). Yet the bias toward government aid prerogatives is also borne out by realities on the ground. Over the course of the conflict, and for entirely different reasons, opposition-controlled Raqqa and Idlib received the least assistance despite having "scored highest on a scale of severity of needs across sectors" (Leenders and Mansour 2018, 225–57).

More broadly, in terms of aid allocation, it "used to be about 50/50, but by 2018 was 80/20" in favor of the government (international humanitarian organization, interview, March 12, 2018). This is not surprising given the progressive losses in opposition-held territory. Yet despite this disparity, an understanding of the impact of humanitarian aid on the Syrian war economy would be incomplete if the focus remained entirely on government-held areas. Even if the proportions differ, armed groups are also guilty of having "obstructed, manipulated and seized humanitarian aid" (Leenders and Mansour 2018, 225–57), and are likewise active participants in the war economy.

External support to opposition groups primarily operating out of Idlib has essentially been for military and humanitarian ends. Military funding and financial backing have been particularly strong from the Gulf region, as well as from "wealthy private funders from Kuwait and Saudi Arabia." As with all data from rebel areas, however, quantifying amounts from Gulf charities and remittances is extremely difficult (international humanitarian organization, interview, March 8, 2018). Also tricky is measuring the outputs of support used for multiple ends. In addition to financing the armed struggle, money has been directed to a "wide selection of projects in opposition areas, such as hospitals, water wells, or bakeries." Combined with more traditional humanitarian aid from international organizations and Syrian expatriates, the potential for misuse is significant (Yazigi 2014).

In the main opposition-held areas of the north, a combination of Damascus-directed aid restrictions, security challenges, and the "inadequacy of UN cross-border and frontline" assistance led most aid organizations to shift the clandestine management and procurement of their operations to southern Turkey (Leenders and Mansour 2018, 225–57). Despite the drawback of receiving unwanted attention from the Turkish authorities, "at least 75 percent of Idlib and Aleppo" are dependent on aid as a source of income, "feeding into everything and arguably prolonging the conflict." In Idlib alone it is estimated that the humanitarian sector contributes "$3.5 million a month" in cash to Tahrir al-Sham (HTS), one of the dominant opposition groups, "out of their total revenue of roughly $10 million a month" (international humanitarian organizations, interviews, March 8 and 12, 2018).

A breakdown of this amount is nearly impossible, because it takes place on so many levels, and there is a significant gap between "suspected and reported diversion." Nevertheless, easily exploitable sectors include beneficiary lists (sometimes referred to as ghost lists, especially through local councils); recruitment and salaries; taxes on the procurement of supplies (non food items [NFI], food, and fuel in particular); the renting of vehicles; and the imposition of contracts in exchange for access. According to those interviewed, medical supplies seem to have been left "relatively alone as items do not regularly appear in local markets." The much-touted third-party monitoring, often the main recourse to supervision, has limitations, however, because such monitors "also play the game" (international humanitarian organizations, interviews, March 8 and12, 2018).

For all the noted elements that have emerged in the transformation of Syria's economy to a war setting, the essential point is that the government's "domination of the business community" means it has an interest in almost all financial exchanges (Humanitarian Access Team, Mercy Corps, pers. comm., March 2018). This is obviously the case where a modicum of central control has been maintained, but it is also true in besieged and hard-to-reach areas. In the protracted sieges of opposition-held territory, fundamental aspects of Syria's war economy are placed in stark relief. Whether "profiteering from cash transfers and currency exchanges" or business monopolies over various items (Sinjab 2017), the grubby interplay of commercial interests surpasses ideological and political disputes.

Government and progovernment forces have relied "time and time again" on siege warfare. The strategy of "siege and starve until submission" has been employed largely because "it works," and is a cost-effective way to "win back territory with minimal cost." But outside military effectiveness, the besieging of opposition enclaves has "evolved from a military tactic into a profitable underground economy" (Ciezadlo 2016; Beehner et al. 2016).[9] And while Syria's war economy has come to dominate the country's economic structures well beyond such enclaves, it is through the use of siege warfare that systemic diversion has been at its most acute.

Crucial to understanding sieges is acknowledging the besieger's objective not only to "defeat the other side" but also for both government and opposition forces to "collude on what enters and exits the area and how," and thus make a fortune in the process (Turkmani et al. 2015). Initially the tactical choice of imposing sieges stemmed from the nature of the conflict. Populated opposition-held parts of the country were surrounded, "ensuring they could not threaten key areas of strategic importance," nor access Damascus proper. This also preserved limited manpower in government forces and prevented viable political alternatives (Todman 2017). As was amply demonstrated in the battles for Homs and Aleppo, civilians and infrastructure were then targeted, and supplies of food and medicine were severely affected (Beehner et al. 2016).

Opposition forces' refusal to surrender resulted in extended stalemates, the last of which were broken in 2018. And as the sieges became entrenched and the war economy grew in both scale and breadth, the use of sieges "became an important element of the regime's survival." Checkpoint duty has been a reward and opportunity for individual soldiers to profit. Traders close to the presidential administration have purchased contracts to trade in specific goods, arguably giving the government incentive to "prolong sieges for financial reasons, making economic payoffs of sieges as vital as their military objectives." Basically, the intertwining of "military and economic benefits" explains the widespread use of siege tactics and their longevity (Todman 2017).

As the duration of sieges began to be counted in years, rebel commanders were forced to spend more time "ensuring access to resources and guarding against threats to their supply lines." Although political leverage was certainly created, in that controlling the amount of goods entering an enclave could "sow enmity among rebels," opportunities to benefit personally from the "lucrative smuggling economy" were significant (Lund 2016). And those businessmen and fixers who successfully "monopolized" certain items or aspects of the siege could similarly profit immensely and gain influence in the area.

For all its underlying good intentions, humanitarian assistance represented a commodity much like anything else entering a besieged area. And even if the procurement of food and fuel were proven the most vulnerable, medical items were not excluded. Aid was therefore undeniably part of a system designed to feed the war economy, with nuances limited to mitigating its most overt abuse.

In the context of captive enclaves, then, the essential aspect to consider for humanitarian actors is that the "cost of a commodity already includes an access fee built into the price." Whether an item is purchased in government-controlled or besieged areas makes no difference in reducing an aid organization's contribution to the war economy. So long as the same middlemen facilitate access on either side of the warring parties, "profits remain distributed to the same key actors" (Humanitarian Access Team, Mercy Corps, pers. comm., March 2018). Amid the very obvious cases of bribery, corruption, looting, and so on, it is easy to lose sight of the broader system in which the vast majority of transactions hold some benefit to the Syrian government.

Due to government-imposed restrictions on aid deliveries, basically the only way for humanitarian organizations to bypass the entire system of war economy was through aid convoys that had been supplied externally to the conflict zone. This is "exactly why the regime is so reluctant to all this process, and also why they prefer a system that is more exploitable" (Free Syrian Army, interview, March 10, 2018). Statistics certainly bear this out. In 2017, authorization was granted for "around 25 percent of requested UN convoys to besieged and hard-to-reach areas." And even then, items were regularly removed, particularly medical supplies. Of the fifty-five convoys that year, only one reached its destination without incident or loss of some cargo (Beals 2018).

Although secondary to the unwitting financing of government and opposition groups, there are other consequences to providing aid to besieged populations. Those who profited from a siege "acquired a vested interest in maintaining it," while armed groups' access to aid in the enclaves could be used to influence the population (Lund 2016). Irrespective of how much wealth was accrued, and as with commercial transactions humanitarian aid certainly influenced the size of the contracts to import items along with the corresponding profit margins, the enclaves invariably collapsed when politically and militarily expedient.

SIEGE ECONOMIES IN PRACTICE: THE EXAMPLE OF EAST GHOUTA

Until its fall to government forces in March 2018, East Ghouta was the most media-exposed although far from the only, example of a besieged population in Syria. The pattern in East Ghouta, repeated elsewhere in besieged and hard-to-reach areas in south and central Syria, provides a microcosm of both the war economy and its capacity to absorb humanitarian aid in a larger system of opportunistic business dealings (Siege Watch 2019).[10] Irrespective of the state of conflict and blockade, "certain pro-government and pro-opposition commanders" have remained connected, "muddling their political and military incentives and complicating any analysis of the situation" (Lund 2016).

With a trapped population and Damascus markets nearby, East Ghouta was an ideal situation for the middlemen described earlier to position themselves profitably. In this regard, Mohieddine Manfoush emerged as an important figure thanks to his close ties with the Syrian government and Jaysh al-Islam. His Manfoush Trading Company established a monopoly on food and fuel being imported into the enclave, with cheap milk and dairy products moving in the opposite direction (D'Alançon 2018). And as the "only trader allowed to bring goods in and out of Syria's largest besieged area," he could manipulate and control prices to a captive market (*Economist* 2017).

Although Wafideen crossing, or "One Million Crossing" for the $5,000 per hour in bribes it was rumored to generate, was the most visible part of the system, significant profits were also generated elsewhere (*Economist* 2017). Fees for moving hard currency into the enclave from aid organizations and the diaspora made their way back to the Manfoush Trading Company before "cash reached its intended recipient, whether that is a hospital, local council office or individual family" (Nassara and Schuster

2017). As profits needed to be spread to all sides, East Ghouta ended up as a "source of monetary support for the regime, but also, paradoxically, for the rebels" (Lund 2016).

Whether government forces held back retaking East Ghouta because it was "more attractive as an economic dairy cow," as some have claimed, is debatable (*Neue Zurcher Zeitung* 2017). What is undeniable is that the "intersection of business and the fighting" has shaped the contours of the conflict, and humanitarians have not escaped unscathed. As one close observer noted, "either you deal with the Manfoushes of this conflict or you do not, but if you do you are absolutely part of it whatever your intention, and aid has clearly abetted one side or another, often both" (international correspondent, interview, March 28, 2018).

AID-RELATED DILEMMAS: THE EXAMPLE OF MÉDECINS SANS FRONTIÈRES

In the internal jargon of the organization, MSF's assistance to besieged enclaves such as East Ghouta has generally taken the form of "distant support." This entails providing medical structures with the financial and locally purchased material means to remain functional (MSF, internal document, "MSF-Reflection Towards More Efficient 'Service Delivery' in Syria" 2016). A central rationale for this approach has been the impossibility of establishing an official presence. By the second year of the conflict, "antiterrorist" legislation had been passed by the government, recognizing only "registered medical facilities" as health structures (MSF, internal document, "The Dynamics of Medical Procurement in Besieged Areas" August 2016). And despite repeated overtures, there was little chance of MSF receiving such recognition. This was articulated publicly in no uncertain terms following the bombing of another MSF-supported hospital in Idlib. Syria's ambassador to the United Nations stated that the "so-called hospital was installed without any prior consultation with the Syrian government by the so-called French network called MSF which is a branch of the French intelligence operating in Syria" (Spencer 2016).

For MSF, the "distant support" model came to be considered a recourse of last resort, a result of extreme needs combined with administrative refusals and a long list of security incidents that made direct intervention impractical or irresponsible. In adopting this model, however, MSF belatedly, and not with a little discomfort, joined long-standing trends in humanitarian assistance in which aid organizations focus on "specific stages of complex supply chains" involving a wide array of partners and contractors (Carbonnier 2015, 58). This is absolutely the case in Syria, where "INGOs generally act as middlemen" (MSF staff, interview, Berlin, March 22, 2018). Basically, humanitarian organizations have "embraced outsourcing and subcontracting" as they move away from the "direct provision of humanitarian aid." The focus instead is on "coordination, fundraising and advocacy" while the actual relief work is carried out by locally based partners (Carbonnier 2015, 58–59).

The approach taken by MSF in East Ghouta and similar enclaves led the organization to develop numerous measures of control. Obvious cases of fraud or looting were generally identified by "crosschecking with local actors, Syrian opposition directorate of health, other local and international NGOs supporting the facilities," and were followed by remedial action (MSF staff, pers. comm., April 2018; MSF, internal documents: "Adra: The Case of Misuse of Funds," February 2015; "Incidents, Transporters, Suppliers," undated; "QNR-CL Investigation," undated). However, the focus on "traditional aid diversion such as bribery and low-level theft" obscured the larger picture. As described, in the Syrian context, war economy refers to a "highly complex, multi-layered system" ensuring that those close to or attached to the presidential administration "benefit from nearly all transactions, to include both locally procured and cross-line humanitarian aid delivery" (Humanitarian Access Team, Mercy Corps, pers. comm., March 2018).

For example, internal MSF analyses note a repeated pattern—evident during the bombing of enclaves—of "hoarding items" by local suppliers, and when the siege tightened "goods were released at ever higher prices." Corruption at checkpoints "reduced the efficiency of such a strategy" and provided a de facto lifeline to trapped civilians, especially as smuggling "provided only minute amounts with respect to their requirements." In other words, "the more corrupt the checkpoint, the lower the siege and the better for the besieged population" (MSF staff, interview, Beirut; MSF, internal documents: "The Dynamics of Medical Procurement"; "The Dynamics of Money Transfer," March 31, 2017).

The result in practical terms was a dramatic increase in costs related to "distant support" projects, particularly over the course of 2017 and 2018, leading up to the fall of East Ghouta. The transfer of money, along with the purchase and transport of material, were all recognized to have played a role, as did the "volatile situation, losses of entry points, hoarding activities and appreciating exchange rates" (MSF, internal document, "Report on Prices: May 2017 to March 2018," March 8, 2018). Most important, however, was the recognition that "all actors and all products and services, not just humanitarian aid," had been targeted. MSF was no less vulnerable than anyone else in attempting to operate in this context (MSF, internal document, "Rapport de visite: 8/2–11/2/2017," February 20, 2017).

THE BROADER AID SYSTEM IN QUESTION

This radical departure from MSF's traditional modus operandi as described above has provoked much internal debate and no consensus over the "appropriateness of indirect programs." Because MSF was able to work only in opposition areas, issues of neutrality were likewise questioned, as was the reliability of information (MSF staff, interview, Beirut; MSF, internal document, "5-Year OCB Response to the Syrian Crisis: Capitalization Work" December 2016). However much as the payment of bribes to get supplies to civilians ignores the fact that such transactions perpetuate the system, it also ignores the system itself. Given the doubts raised about the misuse of aid in the Syrian conflict, it is also relevant to question the degree to which others who structure and finance humanitarian assistance have raised concerns.

The lack of responsibility at all levels of the aid machine, donors included, is striking. One observer aptly described a situation in which "the donors make demands, the NGOs and media bash the UN, the auditors bash the NGOs, and the kaleidoscope of aid agency alliances shifts," and "the international system is starting to look a little like the Syrian conflict" (Parker 2016). Put more succinctly, an uncomfortable compromise transpires, as organizations and their backers attempt to flesh out an operational space while ignoring the broader consequences.

More cynically, it has been claimed that donors "rarely raise questions, and never publicly," because there is "no interest in tarnishing the UN-led aid effort in which they invested so heavily and for which they could not think of an alternative" (Leenders and Mansour 2018, 225–57). Such views are hardly moderated by aid organizations that have decided "once an item crosses the border, it's not my problem" (international humanitarian organization, interview, March 7, 2018). To say that nothing has changed would be an exaggeration, however, because there is discreet but genuine concern about the secondary effects of aid, notably as per the war economy.

Situations such as that described in Idlib are a particular worry, and "donors are anxious" because of groups like HTS being designated as terrorists (international humanitarian organization, interview, 12 March 2018). Indeed, it was in this area that the most significant diversion scandal in opposition-held territory occurred. In 2016, the United States Agency for International Development (USAID) suspended $230 million in funding during a fraud investigation that implicated the major aid actors International Medical Corps, International Rescue Committee, and GOAL. Noting that "corrupt sub-contracting and procurement fraud is undermining vital cross-border relief for desperate Syrians," there was also recognition that "the supply chain involved is big-business" (Slemrod and Parker 2016).

Such investigations, however, can also be viewed as problematic. There is certainly a tendency to shift blame and culpability to aid organizations, who in turn shift it locally (international humanitarian organization, interview, 12 March 2018). There is also a willful ignorance in claiming that "NGOs have to assume responsibility" (international donor, interview, March 9, 2018) rather than the collective aid system, donors included. And the complexity of understanding "cross-border financial flows" exceeds the competencies of most aid organizations. The difficulty of doing so provokes the basic question of whether it is "reasonable" for donors to "transfer the responsibility of political economy and financial analysis to its partners, or treat the risk by being more involved in mitigation" (Beechwood International 2015).

Perhaps the most damning indictment of inadvertent participation in the Syrian war economy comes from within the United Nations itself. In noting the "massive naiveté and irresponsibility" of most humanitarian actors in assuming the broader consequences of aid, as part of the aid system, "donors are as culpable as anyone else" (international humanitarian organization, interview, 12 March 2018). The focus on "traditional war economy threats" of basic diversion and fraud masks the "complexity and pervasiveness" of the Syrian war economy (Humanitarian Access Team, Mercy Corps, pers. comm., March 2018).

HOW IMPORTANT IS HUMANITARIAN AID TO THE SYRIAN WAR ECONOMY?

Answering the above question requires untangling a multitude of views. To one extreme, an observer has emphasized the "responsibility" attached to humanitarian assistance. In this view, aid actors "have played the game" by their unwitting support of the Syrian government or other armed groups and so must bear some responsibility. In a context where the "regime has so many vested interests it is like an octopus, further complicated by non-state actors," the control and diversion of aid is used as a "tool for war ends and profit" (international correspondent, interview, 28 March 2018). Helpfully, the Free Syrian Army adds that while humanitarians contribute "no more than 20 to 25 percent" of armed group funding, directly or indirectly we are "buying from the regime" (Free Syrian Army, interview, 10 March 2018).

Yet a strong element of collective hubris also has long permeated practitioners of humanitarian aid. If humanitarians take credit for the war economy, they "overestimate their own importance." From this perspective, income from humanitarian assistance is minimal compared with other resources. As for the preferred military tactic of the Syrian government, aid cannot contribute to sieges nor their prolongation, because they are "above all about politics." Rather, humanitarian aid contributes by providing "political rather than financial legitimacy to the opposition" (MSF staff, interview, Berlin, 22 March 2018). And given the geopolitical aspects of the conflict, the tendency is for humanitarian aid to "play an even smaller role in its trajectory" (Jihad Yazigi, interview, 22 March 2018).

By narrowly focusing on the importance of aid contributions to the war economy, issues of scale and proportion compared with other resources risk being ignored. Similarly, aid fungibility is relevant to understanding how assistance can "unburden the government of some responsibility," thus freeing up the means to pursue military objectives (Yazigi 2014). UN contracts linked to "regime personalities have benefited both the regime and its militias," in addition to bringing US dollars into the marketplace and "alleviating state responsibility for basic services" (Jihad Yazigi, interview, 22 March 2018). Whether this was essential to the state's survival is debatable, but clearly the provision of assistance, both to the presidential administration and areas under the control of opposition groups, has hardly encouraged investment in services supported by humanitarian organizations.

Toward yet another extreme is the view that "by avoiding politics and claiming neutrality," aid agencies are deceiving themselves. By just setting foot in East Ghouta, "you are perceived as not neutral" and are indirectly "prolonging the conflict." This aspect is largely ignored, given that "organizations are not honest with themselves because they want to remain present at all costs" and certainly not show the "negative side to their activities" (international humanitarian organization, interview, March 12, 2018). Unintended consequences of humanitarian operations in Syria are not limited to questions over participation in the war economy. It also has been argued that "collectively we are making the situation worse in other ways." This includes contributing to the destabilization of any semblance of a health system in opposition areas, with aid organizations supporting "individual structures with an array of protocols"—or indeed competing with one another to provide support (MSF staff, interview, Hatay, March 13, 2018).

Despite the arguments that humanitarian organizations have overestimated their importance, a credible position seems to be "an underestimation of how influential we have become, and there is no doubt that we are contributing to the war economy" (international humanitarian organization, interview, 12 March 2018). Declaring that humanitarian aid should be on the "highest pedestal of moral high ground" rather than part of the "conflict ecosystem" is admittedly naïve and unrealistic (international correspondent, interview, 28 March 2018). Nor does Syria need to lead to an "existential crisis in humanitarianism." Rather, some transparency and "honesty over our failures" would be welcome (international humanitarian organization, interview, 12 March 2018). Until then, perhaps the answer to the question lies elsewhere, between conceited irrelevancy or willful ignorance. Or as an armed actor to the conflict explained, "While the regime is playing with us, you are useful idiots for all sides" (Free Syrian Army, interview, 10 March 2018).

FROM SECURITY TO FINANCIAL RISK—AND THE CHALLENGES AHEAD

Returning to MSF, this last comment implies that the organization walked blindly into a situation with little understanding of the dilemmas and risks of instrumentalization. This hardly reflects the internal discussions and analyses that accompanied the distant support model from its inception. Decisions to "knowingly fund health facilities that buy their drugs from a market" with dramatic markups and questionable quality are not taken lightly (MSF staff, pers. comm., February 20, 2018). Nor is replacing security risks with financial risks, an accountability conundrum impossible to resolve without putting people further at risk.

As we have seen, however, the extensive and understandable focus on controlling resources and limiting adverse consequences has at times blurred the larger question of systemic diversion to which all aid actors in Syria are held hostage to some degree. In MSF's case, choosing to work in Syria required "accepting that we are entering into a war economy," quite possibly at another level than seen elsewhere. This included all the uncomfortable compromises in dealing with "intermediaries that must be paid," knowing full well that many of those intermediaries benefited from the chaos (MSF, internal document, "Rapport de visite: 8/2–11/2/2017," February 20, 2017).

Indeed, an unusual aspect to the Syrian context is the role of businessmen and intermediaries "playing both sides" of the conflict (MSF staff, interview, Beirut, March 9, 2018). Operating out of the "grey zones of politics and the war economy," opportunistic individuals, much as described in East Ghouta, have become wealthy and influential without "registering in the politicized narratives that dominate media coverage of the conflict" (Lund 2016). And with these same middlemen simultaneously supporting "the goals of the regime and opposition forces," a bizarre reinvention of entrepreneurial neutrality has emerged (Abboud 2013). This is all the more striking when compared to the sharp divisions that exist in the aid industry.

With aid organizations essentially divided between those operating out of government and opposition-held territory, there is some credence to concerns over neutrality. Arguably the lower-level middlemen and traders are the most neutral actors in the conflict, profit being the overriding motive in place of humanitarian ideals—the obvious distinction being that those same business actors also have a direct interest in prolonging the conflict, further complicating a resolution and an eventual return to some form of normality.

More broadly, elements of Syria's war economy are likely to maintain their allure even as the region stumbles into a postconflict era. Despite "reconstruction" rhetoric, official support will remain limited. Those countries that might have traditionally carried this burden are essentially on the losing side. And the countries that will have won the war, Russia and Iran, do not have the "financial means to pay for reconstruction" (Jihad Yazigi, interview; Yazigi 2018).[11] Perhaps more fundamentally, after seven years of conflict, there is the basic fact that "marginal returns on a peace economy compared to marginal returns on war economy" have become profoundly disproportionate (international donor, interview, 12 March 2018).

NOTES

1. Despite the obvious negative connotations, there is little academic consensus on the meaning of a war economy when the role of humanitarian aid is included. For the purposes of this chapter, four overlapping categories are used: finance-generating activities that "fund or sustain a war effort"; "survival activities" on the part of the population that can contribute to a conflict; criminal or black-market activities that "flourish under a general climate of impunity generated by the war"; and external relations that connect all these elements to the "global marketplace."

2. Exceptions to these privatization initiatives include "the oil industry, electricity, water, and telephone landlines."

3. "Corruption Perceptions Index," Transparency International, 2010 and 2019, https://www.transparency.org/en/cpi#.

4. Turkey and Saudi Arabia had a combined official trade with Syria of $3.6 billion in 2010 compared with $316 million from Iran.
5. For example, during the six-month siege of the government military base Wadi Deif in 2013, opposition commanders took bribes from the army to allow food supplies to be sent to its own men inside.
6. By the end of 2013, food imports, not under sanction, were a significant source of profit. "A cargo of 100,000 tonnes of wheat attracts at least a $3 million to $4 million mark-up," and "sugar deliveries carry a 5 to 7 percent premium, also meaning millions of dollars in the margins."
7. More precisely, in addition to the MoFA, the Ministry of Local Administration, SARC, and Syria Trust are key entities in the government control of the aid system.
8. OCHA citation taken from "Aleppo Is Screwed. Thanks Everyone." (See References.)
9. Opposition forces also have used siege tactics, notably in Foue and Kefraya.
10. In addition to East Ghouta, by mid-2013 long-term sieges were entrenched in southern Damascus suburbs, parts of West Ghouta, northern Homs, and the Old City of Homs.
11. It is interesting to note that "Russia has actually made profit out of killing Syrians, through the various export deals won by its arms industry," but provided little direct aid. The same can be said of Iran aside from oil supplies and lines of credit.

REFERENCES

Abboud, Samer. 2017. "The Economics of War and Peace in Syria: Stratification and Factionalization in the Business Community." In *Arab Politics Beyond the Uprisings*, edited by Thanassis Cambanis and Michael Wahid Hanna. Century Foundation. https://tcf.org/content/report/economics-war-peace-syria/

Abboud, Samer. 2013. "Syria's Business Elite: Between Political Alignment and Hedging Their Bets." German Institute for International and Security Affairs, Stiftung Wissenschaft und Politik. Berlin.

Beals, Emma. 2018. "UN Shelved 2017 Reforms to Syria Aid Response." *New Humanitarian*, February 26, 2018. https://www.thenewhumanitarian.org/feature/2018/02/26/exclusive-un-shelved-2017-reforms-syria-aid-response.

Beechwood International. 2015. *Technical Assessment: Humanitarian Use of Hawala in Syria*. London: Beechwood International.

Beehner, Lionel M., Michael T. Jackson, and Benedetta Berti. 2016. "Modern Siege Warfare: How It Is Changing Counterinsurgency." *Foreign Affairs*, December 7, 2016.

Carbonnier, Gilles. 2015. *Humanitarian Economics*. London: Hurst & Company.

Chulov, Martin, and Emma Beals. 2014. "Aid Group Mercy Corps Forced to Close Damascus Operations." *Guardian*, May 23, 2014.

Ciezadlo, Annia. 2016. "The Siege Sector: Why Starving Civilians Is Big Business." *New Humanitarian*, August 11, 2016. https://deeply.thenewhumanitarian.org/syria/articles/2016/08/10/my-days-in-damascus-entry-3-the-post-revolution-generation.

D'Alançon, François. 2018. "Syrie: Al Wafadine, un check-point cogéré par le régime et Jaych al-Islam." *La Croix*, March 16, 2018.

Economist. 2017. "Dairy Godfathers: Syria's New War Millionaires." *Economist*, June 1, 2017. https://www.economist.com/middle-east-and-africa/2017/06/01/syrias-new-war-millionaires.

Hopkins, Nick, and Emma Beals. 2016a. "How Assad Regime Controls UN Aid Intended for Syria's Children." *Guardian*, August 29, 2016. https://www.theguardian.com/world/2016/aug/29/how-assad-regime-controls-un-aid-intended-for-syrias-children.

Hopkins, Nick, and Emma Beals. 2016b. "UN Pays Tens of Millions to Assad Regime under Syria Aid Programme." *Guardian*, August 29, 2016. https://www.theguardian.com/world/2016/aug/29/un-pays-tens-of-millions-to-assad-regime-syria-aid-programme-contracts.

Leenders, Reinoud. 2016. "UN's \$4bn Aid Effort in Syria Is Morally Bankrupt." *Guardian*, August 29, 2016. https://www.theguardian.com/world/commentisfree/2016/aug/29/uns-4bn-aid-effort-in-syria-is-morally-bankrupt.

Leenders, Reinoud, and Kholoud Mansour. 2018. "Humanitarianism, State Sovereignty and Authoritarian Regime Maintenance in the Syrian War." *Political Science Quarterly* 133 (2): 225–57.

Lund, Aron. 2016. *Into the Tunnels: The Rise and Fall of Syria's Rebel Enclave in the Eastern Ghouta*. Century Foundation. Consulted online: https://tcf.org/content/report/into-the-tunnels/?agreed=1

Lund, Aron. 2018. *The Factory: A Glimpse into Syria's War Economy*. Century Foundation. Consulted online: https://tcf.org/content/report/factory-glimpse-syrias-war-economy/

Nassara, Alaa, and Justin Schuster. 2017. "Bribes, Graft and the Cost of Moving Cash in Syria's War Economy." *Syria Direct*, July 27, 2017.

Neue Zurcher Zeitung. 2017. "Die Barbarei der Kriegswirtschaft: Der nicht enden wollende Krieg in Syrien wird von seinen Akteuren auch durch Profitstreben am Leben erhalten." *Neue Zurcher Zeitung* (internal translation), October 11, 2017.

Parker, Ben. 2016. "Aleppo Is Screwed. Thanks Everyone." *New Humanitarian*, July 29, 2016.

Saul, Jonathan. 2013. "Assad Allies Profit from Syria's Lucrative Food Trade." *Reuters*, November 14, 2013. https://www.reuters.com/article/syria-food/exclusive-assad-allies-profit-from-syrias-lucrative-food-trade-idUKL5N0IZ4MX20131114.

Shanahan, Roger. 2018. "The Trouble Telling Aid Workers and Foreign Fighters Apart." *BBC*, March 15, 2018. https://www.bbc.com/news/world-middle-east-42861695.

Sherlock, Ruth. 2013. "Syria Dispatch: From Band of Brothers to Princes of War." *Telegraph*, November 30, 2013. https://www.telegraph.co.uk/news/worldnews/middleeast/syria/10485970/Syria-dispatch-from-band-of-brothers-to-princes-of-war.html.

Siege Watch. 2019. *Final Report—Out of Sight, Out of Mind: The Aftermath of Syria's Sieges*. Siege Watch, March 6, 2019.

Sinjab, Lina. 2017. "How Syria's War Economy Propels the Conflict." Chatham House, July 2017.

Slemrod, Anni, and Ben Parker. 2016. "US Probe into Turkey-Syria Aid Corruption Deepens." *New Humanitarian (formerly IRIN)*, May 9, 2016.

Sparrow, Annie. 2018. "How UN Humanitarian Aid Has Propped Up Assad: Syria Shows the Need for Reform." *Foreign Affairs*, September 20, 2018.

Spencer, Richard. 2016. "'Médecins Sans Frontières Run by French Intelligence,' Says Assad Regime." *Telegraph*, February 17, 2016.

Todman, Will. 2017. "The Resurgence of Siege Warfare." *CCAS Newsmagazine*, Fall/Winter 2017.

Tokmajyan, Armenak. 2016. *The War Economy in Northern Syria*. Aleppo Project, December 2016.

Turkmani, Rim, Ali A. K. Ali, Mary Kaldor, and Vesna Bojicic-Dzelilovic. 2015. *Countering the Logic of the War Economy in Syria; Evidence from Three Local Areas*. London: London School of Economics and Political Science.

World Bank. 2016. *Syria's Economic Outlook*. World Bank, Fall 2016.

Yazigi, Jihad. 2018. "Opinion: No Reconstruction for Syria." February 14, 2018. https://jihadyazigi.com/2018/02/.

Yazigi, Jihad. 2014. "Syria's War Economy." European Council on Foreign Relations, April 2014.

CHAPTER 6

Endless Siege

The Chain of Complicity in Syrian Suffering

JONATHAN WHITTALL

Siege is most commonly understood as a military tactic of encirclement of an opposition in order to force a defeat. This most basic definition, however, does not capture the multiple ways in which civilians in conflict experience besiegement.

In Syria, siege means being encircled by armed forces, starved, denied access to medical treatment or food, and prevented from fleeing violence. For Syria as a whole, siege means borders being sealed. It means being shot at or abused by border guards while trying to cross to safety. It means having no legal status in neighboring countries, where mobility and residence for Syrians, and other refugees, is restricted. For refugees attempting to reach Europe, siege means running the dangerous gauntlet to enter "fortress Europe." It means navigating a policy-made obstacle course of physical and administrative barriers and risking lives on an overcrowded boat to cross the Mediterranean, in some cases while being chased by EU-funded Libyan coast guards wanting to take you back to a country at war (MSF 2016a; Ponthieu 2015). It means being stranded and contained on a Greek island while being used as a political bargaining chip, traded for multibillion Euro deals such as that struck between the European Union and Turkey. It means being unable to pay for food or access medical supplies due to economic sanctions imposed on an entire country.

Jonathan Whittall, *Endless Siege* In: *Everybody's War*. Edited by: Jehan Bseiso, Michiel Hofman, and Jonathan Whittall, Oxford University Press. © Médecins Sans Frontières 2021. DOI: 10.1093/oso/9780197514641.003.0007

Understanding besiegement from the perspective of the besieged broadens the notion of siege. Siege follows Syrian civilians from within their countries to the places they seek refuge. It systematically weakens their infrastructure of survival. The effects extend far beyond an army's stated objectives of military encirclement, and those involved in implementing besiegement extend far beyond the direct parties to a conflict. Political opponents otherwise separated by interests and ideologies appear united in their use of siege tactics. There is a chain of complicity, in generating human suffering and exploiting it, from Syria to its neighbors and from Europe to its international allies. Humanitarian aid, including both its denial and provision, has been weaponized and turned against Syrians by those implementing a siege.

To expose the real intentions and impact of siege, we need to explore how the tactic is used in military doctrine, how the understanding of siege can be broadened, and how this applies to the case of Syria. From this understanding, we can comprehend the true impact of besiegement.

SIEGE IN MILITARY DOCTRINE: THE CASE OF BEIRUT IN 1982

We most commonly associate military siege with a city. In the post–Cold War era, Sarajevo marked one of the most iconic moments of siege. Later, Grozny featured as a symbol of the brutality of siege tactics. More recently, Aleppo, Eastern Ghouta, and Mosul have been vivid illustrations of this age-old military tactic.

The example used by the United States, in its Army Field Manual 3-06 for training on urban operations, is Beirut in 1982 (Urban Operations 2006): Palestinian and Syrian forces, along with the civilian population in the western part of the city, came under a brutal Israeli siege. For over a month, Israeli forces controlled the supplies in and out of West Beirut. They cut water and electricity, conducted ground offensives to take territory, and carried out major air offensives to weaken the Palestinian Liberation Organization (PLO) and its supporters. Ultimately, the PLO left the city. This came days after a massive death toll of civilians caused by an Israeli airstrike. "The Israelis attacked from multiple directions, segmented West Beirut into pieces, and then destroyed each individually," the US field manual says (Urban Operations 2006, A-21). This case study is the only example of siege the manual cites, and is intended as an approach to learn from, to replicate. No mention is made of the immense civilian toll of the siege. Rather, the manual states that "the tactical plan was sound," and the siege was both a political and a military success (Urban Operations 2006, A-21).

A primary tactic used by Israeli forces was that of psychological warfare:

> The IDF used passive measures, such as leaflet drops and loudspeaker broadcasts. They used naval bombardment to emphasize the totality of the isolation of Beirut. To maintain high levels of stress, to deny sleep, and to emphasize their combat power, the IDF used constant naval, air, and artillery bombardment. They even employed sonic booms from low-flying aircraft to emphasize the IDF's dominance, a tactic that has continued in the besiegement of Gaza. These efforts helped to convince the PLO that the only alternative to negotiation on Israeli terms was complete destruction. (Urban Operations 2006, A-20)

When it came to the provision of aid, the US field manual states, "since essential services were under Israeli command, and had been since the beginning of the siege, the Israelis had the ability to easily restore these resources to West Beirut as soon as they adopted the cease-fire." The deprivation of access to essential services was therefore an integral component of the strategy to force surrender and to deny any "benefit" to the enemy.

The manual argues that the siege on Beirut succeeded because the "PLO's military situation became untenable before the Israeli political situation did" (Urban Operations 2006, A-16). Essentially, a military victory was never in question for the Israeli forces at the time. What was in question was whether they could "sustain military operations politically in the face of international and domestic opposition" (Urban Operations 2006, A-16).

The PLO eventually evacuated the city. By giving the PLO a "way out," the US manual argues, the Israeli forces were successful in achieving the final objective of their siege.

This case study demonstrates that at the core of the siege tactic is to show to those trapped within the siege that their choices are either complete destruction or surrender. In Beirut, though the siege's stated target was the PLO, the pressure placed on the civilian population was inextricably linked. In siege there is also a strong principle of deterrence, the tactic demonstrating the harm that can come without surrender. The attackers limit access to life-saving supplies, carry out "shock and awe" military operations, keep the population and fighters under a constant state of stress, and then allow those under siege a final escape route, before the besieging party's brutal tactics are denounced in the court of public opinion.

Siege is the opposite of the counterinsurgency tactic of winning "hearts and minds," also known as "stabilization," which dominated much of the military doctrine of the early 2000s. In "hearts and minds" operations, services are provided to the population to engender their support. In siege-based counterinsurgencies, services are deprived from a population, to punish them for their support of an opponent.

BEYOND THE MILITARY TACTIC OF SIEGE

Examining the military use of siege, as outlined in the US war manual, is not sufficient to understanding the full extent of modern siege warfare and the entirety of ways in which people are placed under blockade. Many of these siege tactics also are used in pursuit of political objectives that in modern times are increasingly defined by states' antiterrorism and antimigration policies.

In their paper, "The Strategic Logic of Sieges in Counterinsurgencies," Lionel M. Beehner, Benedetta Berti, and Michael T. Jackson define a siege as "any attempt by an adversary to control access into and out of a town, neighborhood, or other terrain of strategic significance to achieve a military or political objective" (Beehner et al. 2017, 78). It is in this way that I consider the tactic of siege to extend from military encirclement to include the closure of borders; the administrative obstacles placed on people's ability to leave a conflict environment; and the economic suffocation of opponents for military ends. These all represent attempts to control "terrain of strategic significance." This terrain extends from pieces of land with military importance to include refugees and political enemies. The closure of borders, deterrence measures, administrative hurdles, and sanctions are designed to encircle and entrap—to undermine a population's means of survival so they will surrender to the demands of those who have placed them under siege.

Siege warfare is not necessarily unlawful. In fact, "Siege warfare remains lawful under contemporary law," the human rights scholar Beth Van Schaack writes, "so long as it is directed only at combatants and those directly participating in hostilities, and only in so far as other provisions of the law of war are adhered to—a major challenge when both combatants and civilians are dependent on the same necessities" (Van Schaack 2016).

Based on these considerations, it seems almost impossible for modern-day military and political siege tactics to be considered legal. To starve the enemy inevitably means starving the civilian population, which amounts to a war crime. Counterterrorism doctrine has found a way around this, however. The definitions of "civilian" and "combatant" have been deliberately blurred, eroding the notion of what makes a civilian and expanding the possibility of lawful siege to include entire populations deemed to be enemies, national security risks, and forces of destabilization (Bouchet-Saulnier and Whittall 2018; Whittall 2016). The sociologist Lisa Hajjar refers to the ability of the United States in the so-called war on terror to "prosecute a territorially unbounded war against an evolving cast of enemies" (Hajjar 2019). Hajjar, in her article, "Israel as Innovator in Normalizing Extreme Violence," points out:

> The counterterrorism paradigm of "with us or against us" in which the latter—and all that is proximate to it—is regarded as targetable upends the important distinction in international humanitarian law (IHL) between civilians and combatants and inflates the norm of proportionality to justify indiscriminate violence. This paradigm is the dominant strategic approach in the US "war on terror" and Israel's "war model" approach in the Occupied Territories, as well as among regimes like Syria and Saudi Arabia." (Hajjar, 2016)

The geographer Derek Gregory argues that the war on terror in Afghanistan and Iraq marked the beginning of an "everywhere war," which he describes as a "conceptual and material project" (Gregory 2011, 239). He divides this project into three elements. First, "war has become the pervasive matrix within which social life is constituted"; second, he points out how US military doctrine has shifted to define war as taking place not on a "battlefield," but in an all-encompassing "battle-space" with "no front or back and where everything becomes the site of permanent war"; and third, this war extends to the "borderlands where the United States and its allies now conduct their military operations" (Gregory 2011, 239).

"Everywhere war" posits that territorial control has become irrelevant. In the everywhere war, opponents are "extra-territorial" and constantly on the move. "Within this warscape," Gregory writes, "military and paramilitary violence could descend at any moment without warning, and within it precarious local orders were constantly forming and re-forming" (Gregory 2011, 239). Syria demonstrates how modern-day forms of siege are carried out in this "battle-space."

SURRENDER OR DIE

In Syria, neighborhoods started falling under siege by the Syrian army in mid-2012. Checkpoints and snipers were placed around communities as a way to regulate people's movement and the flow of essential goods in and out of areas that had come under control of the armed opposition. In

2013, these sieges spread to include the surrounding areas of Damascus and parts of Homs (Szybala et al. 2019, 16).

Based on the United Nation's definition of a besieged area—as a place "surrounded by armed actors with the sustained effect that humanitarian assistance cannot regularly enter, and civilians, the sick and wounded cannot regularly exit"—during the course of the Syrian war, it has been estimated that at least 1.45 million people have lived under long-term besiegement (Szybala et al. 2019).

Beehner, Berti, and Jackson argue that for a siege to be effective, two factors must be met: "First, the counterinsurgency must be willing to use overwhelming force, which includes indiscriminate violence or scorched earth tactics. Second, there must be a forceful military intervention on behalf of the besieger by an outside power" (Beehner, Berti, and Jackson 2017, 80). This is certainly the case for Syria, whereas it may not be the case if the besieger is a superpower. The authors argue that without the support of an outside power to tip the balance, "the siege effectively becomes a protracted war of attrition that favors the side with sufficient will and resources to outlast the other" (Beehner, Berti, and Jackson 2017, 80).

In Syria, government forces very clearly adopted this approach; demonstrations of their willingness to use overwhelming force were regularly on display. Although reliable sources are hard to find, some estimate that up to seventy thousand barrel bombs were dropped over Syria up until 2017 (SNHR 2017). Barrel bombs, sometimes referred to as "flying IEDs," are improvised explosives literally packed into a barrel together with shrapnel. Their first reported use was by the Israeli army in 1948, and later, the US army deployed them in Vietnam. These low-cost, high-impact weapons have been used repeatedly in Syria against populations under siege—though in some instances the areas subjected to these shock-and-awe bombing campaigns were able to withstand the pressure to surrender.

In the siege of Aleppo, Beehner et al. point out that the Syrian government did not have the capacity to wage a ground offensive to retake the whole of Eastern Aleppo: "With about 25,000 troops initially, the regime lacked the material strength to occupy the area and struggled to take and to hold territory, especially in this dense urban terrain, without sustaining high casualties and carrying out an extensive house-to-house counterinsurgency campaign" (Beehner, Berti, and Jackson 2017, 82).

Instead, the siege on the city cut off the area from access to basic services. But military progress was slow. It was the increased involvement of Russian air power after December 2015, combined with Iranian and Hezbollah ground forces, that tipped the balance of power to the Syrian government's favor (UNGA 2017).

The Syrian army also has used siege to prevent the opposition from asserting any form of legitimate governance over the areas it has controlled. In addition, siege warfare, together with the destruction of infrastructure and services, has obstructed the opposition's ability to govern or to create viable alternatives to the Syrian government (Jackson, Beehner, and Berti 2016).

Coercive negotiations took place in all areas under siege throughout the war in Syria. But it was Russian involvement in Syria that resulted in the surrendering of entire areas to government control. In 2016 and 2017, a series of "local reconciliation agreements" were reached. These agreements resulted in the forced displacement of armed groups and civilians into northern parts of Syria (most notably Idlib).

Foreign military actors, through their defense or intelligence services, were often directly involved in these negotiations, clearly as a way to demonstrate to the opposition the extent to which the balance of power had tipped in favor of the Syrian government (Adleh and Favier 2017). Talks would take place amid a tightening of the siege. When these talks stalled, there would be an intensification of strikes on the besieged zone. "In essence," Amnesty International found, "the deals have enabled the government to reclaim control of territory by first starving and then removing inhabitants who rejected its rule" (Amnesty International 2017).

Throughout the use of siege tactics in the Syria war, the denial and restoration of access to basic and essential services made up an essential component of the Syrian government's strategy. In the case of Eastern Ghouta, the siege lasted for a total of five years before it was lifted through a reconciliation process. The United Nations (UN) Security Council has passed a multitude of resolutions on the war in Syria, including a call for the cessation of all sieges and the denunciation of the use of starvation of civilians as a method of combat.

Yet it was not only the Syrian army, with the backing of Russian air power and Iranian and Hezbollah ground forces, that made use of siege. The Syrian opposition also besieged towns—though admittedly far fewer—across the country. In the battle against the Islamic State (IS) in Syria and Iraq, the United States used significant air power against civilians trapped alongside IS fighters in areas under siege by local ground forces. Between September 2014 and March 2020, the death toll from the obliteration of these areas by US air power amounted to fourteen thousand people, of whom thirty-eight hundred were estimated to be civilians (Syrian Observatory for Human Rights 2020). In comparison, it is estimated that Russian airstrikes killed twenty thousand people in Syria, of which eighty-six hundred were civilians (Syrian Observatory for Human Rights 2020). These numbers are surely imperfect measurements. But they do indicate that the use of US air power was not insignificant in its impact on people living under siege in Syria—indeed, that the US bombardment was just as brutal as that of the Russians. The difference is a political and not a military one; that is, who is considered a terrorist. For the United States, it was IS; for the Russians, it was the broader Syrian armed opposition.

Throughout the Syrian war, siege and the military operations used alongside it have been justified on the grounds of fighting terrorists. Within this "war on terror" environment, the "with us or against us" approach has resulted in entire communities being designated part of a criminalized enemy, justifying indiscriminate attack, including the tactic of siege. In the context of contemporary counterterrorism operations, it is therefore more useful to understand Gregory's "everywhere war" as being about an "everybody enemy."

In Syria, the form of siege experienced by the population was by definition indiscriminate, because it affected everyone regardless of whether they were a combatant. Although the siege was applied with a "surrender or die" level of intensity, the population was never in a position to surrender—only the combatants could do that. This doesn't seem to have affected the way in which the tactic was used, which only reinforces that everyone under siege was considered an enemy, and the weakening of their means of survival the ultimate objective. Once these vulnerabilities were generated on a mass scale, they were exploited for political and military gain.

BORDERS CLOSED

Over 5.6 million people have fled Syria as refugees into neighboring countries and farther abroad (UNHCR 2020b). As of 2018, this number was almost double those trapped in areas under siege or in "hard to reach" areas inside Syria (UNHCR 2020b). But those who have tried or managed to leave the country have encountered a type of siege being imposed on Syrians occupying the transnational battlespace: closed borders and policy obstacles to their survival in neighboring countries.

A wave of refugees entered neighboring countries in 2013. By March 2015, Syria's neighbors had closed their borders to the country. Although Turkey took in over three million Syrian refugees and provided them with temporary protection, its borders were closed in 2015, and in 2018 Turkish guards along the Syrian border were accused of shooting refugees fleeing the war in Idlib (HRW 2018). In Jordan, approximately 1.8 million Syrian refugees entered the country before the borders were closed.

Jordan's border closure resulted in tens of thousands of people being trapped in a no-man's land at the Rukban and Hadalat border crossings known as "The Berm." One report noted: "In October 2015, 5,000 people were stuck at the border area, however within two months this figure had increased to 14,300 people. While over the course of 2016, the situation got steadily worse and, by the end of the year, the figure stood at 85,000. . . . The UN estimates that four out of five of these displaced people are women and children" (Hajžmanová 2017).

The justification for implementing the entrapment of an "undesirable" refugee population was once again the threat of terrorism, stemming from a 2016 attack on a Jordanian military post in Rukhban. According to the King of Jordan, "Such heinous terrorist acts will only make us more determined to carry on with our fight against terrorism and its groups who plotted in the dark against the men who protect the country and its borders" (Black 2016).

A few months later, in September 2016, Turkey launched Operation Euphrates Shield in the area of Jarablus, ostensibly to prevent Kurdish forces (whom Turkey designates as terrorists) in the northeast of Syria connecting with other areas to the west, such as Afrin. Turkey also claimed that the creation of a "safe zone" would enable the delivery of humanitarian assistance. "The promised humanitarian services however were not widely provided throughout the zone," a Médecins Sans Frontières (MSF) analysis found (Sidahmed 2017). This illustrated that the primary purpose of these safe zones was "to avoid any more refugees leaving Syria and creating spaces where existing refugees are encouraged back into the country in conflict that they tried to flee" (Sidahmed 2017).

Though closed borders and safe zones are obvious manifestations of the hostility or unwelcoming attitude of neighboring countries to Syrian refugees, there are those who have managed to pass this obstacle. Some arrived in neighboring countries prior to 2015, while others were smuggled across porous borders. Border closures often have loopholes for the wealthy.

What the closed border represents—a deterrence—is carried over into the policy approach to refugees in neighboring countries. Syrians who have managed to cross into neighboring countries have faced hostile policies that have been a major obstacle to achieving safety.[1] In Lebanon, writes Maja Janmyr, a professor of international migration law, the country "is neither party to the 1951 Convention relating to the status of refugees, nor does it have any national legislation dealing with refugees" (Janmyr 2016).

This legal vacuum was filled in 2014, when the Lebanese council of ministers adopted a policy on Syrian refugees. The policy aimed to decrease the number of Syrians in the country "by reducing access to territory and encouraging return to Syria" (Janmyr 2016). Through this dual approach of closing borders and implementing a series of measures to deter Syrian asylum seekers, the second layer of siege was reinforced behind the closed borders of Lebanon. As a result, Syrians in Lebanon faced similar choices to those under siege within Syria: surrender and leave, or stay and starve.

In 2014, Human Rights Watch (HRW) counted forty-five local municipalities that had imposed curfews on Syrian refugees in Lebanon (HRW 2014). According to HRW: "Such curfews violate international human rights law and appear to be illegal under Lebanese law. Municipal police enforce many of the curfews but Human Rights Watch also received information about the creation of local vigilante groups to enforce curfews, raising concerns about abuses."

Early in the Syrian war, as refugees started crossing the border, Lebanon banned the construction of permanent structures to house them. This ban has subsequently been used to justify the demolition of homes built by Syrians and the forced return of Syrians to a country still at war. In 2019, Middle East Eye reported that "over 5,600 structures housing Syrian refugees were destroyed, following a decision from Lebanon's military-affiliated Higher Defence Council determining that the concrete-based structures are illegal" (Chehayeb 2019). This came after an earlier decision by the Higher Defense Council that "'semi-permanent structures' built by Syrian refugees using materials other than timber and plastic sheeting in informal camps must be deconstructed" (Terre des Hommes et al. 2019).

These measures have been put in place to ensure the temporary nature of Syrians' presence in neighboring countries. And further measures have been added to underscore the transitory nature of their stay. In Lebanon, for instance, the registration of refugees by the United Nations High Commissioner for Refugees (UNHCR) was suspended in 2015 at the request of Lebanese authorities. According to UNHCR, "Admission to Lebanon is currently restricted to those who can provide valid identity documents and proof that their stay in Lebanon fits into one of the approved reasons for entry. Seeking refuge in Lebanon is not among the valid reasons for entry" (UNHCR 2020a).

In addition, residency regulations introduced by the Lebanese government required all Syrians who managed to enter the country legally to pay the often out-of-reach fee of USD$200 per year in order to stay. They were also required to present "valid identification and an entry slip obtained at the border, submit a housing pledge confirming their place of residence, and provide two photographs stamped by a Lebanese local official. To maintain residency, Syrians not registered with UNHCR have to provide a 'pledge of responsibility' signed by a Lebanese national or registered entity to sponsor an individual or family" (HRW 2017).

As a result of these extreme measures, it is estimated that more than half a million unregistered Syrian refugees are living in Lebanon, in legal limbo—unable to access essential assistance, deprived of adequate housing, and at risk of arrest and deportation (HRW 2017). Nizar Saghieh, a lawyer and human rights activist, has referred to Lebanon's policy approach toward Syrian refugees as "manufacturing vulnerability" (Saghieh 2015).

Palestinian refugees from Syria have been a particularly vulnerable group in neighboring countries. Jordan closed its border to Palestinian refugees from Syria early in the conflict, and Lebanon followed suit. Palestinian refugees were subjected to even harsher entry requirements to Lebanon than Syrians and were not allowed to benefit from any "humanitarian clause" that existed for Syrians. The Lebanese policy toward Palestinian refugees goes "so far as to employ discriminatory measures against the refugees, some of which verge on collective punishment" (Saghieh 2015). This approach to Palestinians pre-dates the Syrian war and paved the way for the Lebanese state's response to Syrian refugees.

In 2019, the Lebanese authorities began implementing their threats to deport Syrians from the country. "In just one month," a report in *Foreign Policy* said, "301 Syrians were summarily deported as Lebanese security agencies implemented an official decision to send back anyone who entered the country illegally after April 24" (Vohra 2019a). Around the same time, Turkey began its own campaign to return Syrians and to remove undocumented Syrians from Istanbul (Vohra 2019b).

SINK OR SWIM

A further extension of the conditions of siege facing Syrians is encountered on their journey to Europe. Considering Europe's current political climate, it does not take a huge stretch of the imagination to see how refugees are being portrayed as an enemy population. Hungary's prime minister has said that if Europe does not take a tougher stand against migrants, "Europe will no longer belong to Europeans" (Walt 2019). Matteo Salvini, the former interior minister of Italy, has referred to migrants as "terrorists" and described dealing with migration as a process of "mass cleaning, street by street." Salvini has referred to migrants arriving by boat to Italy as "delinquents and terrorists" who have gone on to "commit massacres in other European countries." According to Salvini: "Our policy of blocking illegal immigration in Italy is at the service of all of Europe, France, Spain, Germany and Brussels. They give lessons, but the serious policies of both Hungary and Italy save them" (Monella and Amiel 2019). Ursula von der

Leyen, the Head of the European Union Commission, has praised Greece for being "Europe's shield" against migrants (BBC 2020). In Austria, the Interior Ministry renamed refugee reception centers "departure centers," signaling just how unwelcome refugees are (Schultheis 2019). In a speech promoting his model of "Christian democracy," Viktor Orban, the prime minister of Hungary, declared that "liberal democracy is pro-immigration, while Christian democracy is anti-immigration."

By categorizing migrants as "terrorists," European leaders have sought to strip them of their rights to assistance. As the scholars Neve Gordon and Nicola Perugini have pointed out:

> In several countries, the humanitarian approach used to manage the influx of migrants has been increasingly combined with a military one, with some governments waging a war on migrants. In this process, civilians who try to cross political borders are constituted as legitimate targets of military violence— people whose lives do not matter and can be rendered killable. And when life does not matter, surely death too is perceived as inconsequential. (Perugini and Gordon 2018)

A core feature of Europe's migration policy is to prevent the "enemy" from reaching its shores in the first place. Europe's policy has "focused on fortifying borders, developing ever more sophisticated surveillance and tracking of people, and increasing deportations while providing ever fewer legal options for residency despite ever greater need," one report found. "This has led many forcibly displaced persons unable to enter Europe legally and forced into ever more dangerous routes to escape violence and conflict" (Akkerman 2018).

Refugees are essentially besieged through policies that expand Europe's borders outward to prevent refugees from reaching its shores. Through this externalization of borders, proxy forces—in the form of neighboring or transit countries—are used to ensure the "enemy" is kept out. Neighboring countries to Europe are expected, and often compensated handsomely, to play the role of European border guards. Many of these countries, including Libya, Turkey, and Sudan, are either ravaged by war or the spill-over effects of war.

Europe has developed policy tools to ensure this externalization, primarily in the form of massive economic aid with significant border control strings attached.

> This includes collaboration with third countries in terms of accepting deported persons, training of their police and border officials, the development of extensive biometric systems, and donations of equipment including helicopters,

patrol ships and vehicles, surveillance and monitoring equipment. While many projects are done through the European Commission, a number of individual member states, such as Spain, Italy and Germany also take a lead in funding and supporting border externalisation efforts through bilateral agreements with non-EU-countries. (Akkerman 2018)

In many instances this aid is provided to states that have poor track records in terms of refugee protection. Clearly this is not a concern for Europe, considering its own dismal track record on refugee protection: the conditions that refugees and migrants are subjected to on their arrival in Europe are the result of clear policies to generate misery as a deterrent to other migrants.

More than a million refugees have reached the Greek islands since 2015. Those who remain on the island are essentially trapped in overcrowded and squalid conditions, amounting to inhumane and degrading treatment. They are caught in an uncertain holding pattern; some have been or will be sent back to Turkey under the deal signed between the European Union and Turkey in 2016.

This EU deal with Turkey dealt with refugees as though they were bargaining chips. For every refugee who managed to reach Europe's shores, it was expected that another one would be sent back from Greece to Turkey. According to Aurelie Ponthieu from MSF, "This crude calculation reduces people to mere numbers, denying them humane treatment and discarding their right to seek protection in Europe. These people are not numbers, but men, women, children and families. Around 88 percent of those using this route are coming from refugee producing countries, and more than half of them are women and children" (Ponthieu 2016).

At another entry point to Europe, on the border between Hungary and Serbia, Elisabeth Zerofsky wrote in *The New Yorker*, there is a thirteen-foot-tall electric razor-wire fence. "The fence, which is monitored by drones and by soldiers, is equipped with heat sensors and loudspeakers that issue grave warnings in English, Arabic, and Farsi that attempting to cross the border is a crime" (Zerofsky 2019).

On the Mediterranean Sea, European states have supported the Libyan coast guard in preventing migrant boats from leaving Libya, and in intercepting and pushing them back. The Italian state has made the running of independent search-and-rescue boats on the Mediterranean Sea a criminal offense, even though Italy has a limited and insufficient search-and-rescue capacity. As a result, thousands of people are drowning in the mass graveyard of the Mediterranean Sea.

Those returned to Libya face abhorrent conditions (OHCHR 2018). Migrants transiting through Libya are extorted, beaten, humiliated, denied access to basic and life-saving assistance, and placed in inhuman detention facilities where they are tortured. If they manage to make it onto a boat to Europe, they risk drowning at sea, being suffocated in an overcrowded boat, or being intercepted and turned back to their tormentors in Libya (OHCHR 2018).

In 2014 and 2015, the majority of the people crossing from Libya were from Syria, whereas that is less the case today. Migrants come from Afghanistan, Sudan, Eritrea, Ivory Coast, and other sub-Saharan African countries, and all are equally vulnerable and exploited in their search for safety and opportunity. For Syrians who reach Libya, the EU-funded and maintained systematic assault on human dignity represents one of the most brutal implementations of the denial of their right to safety.

Indeed, a chain of complicity in Syrians' suffering exists, from those under siege in their own country to those abused on the borders of Europe.

SUFFOCATED BY SANCTIONS

Siege warfare is concerned not only with the control of population movement, but also—as we have seen in each experience of siege facing Syrians—with the control of access to resources. A form of siege is asserted on the Syrian government and its institutions through sanctions that hamper its ability to sustain basic services to its population. In 1999, Joy Gordon, whose work focuses on human and economic rights, referred to the sanctions regime on Iraq as a "modern-day equivalent of siege warfare" (Gordon 1999b). The journalist Patrick Cockburn, in a scathing article on why sanctions should be considered war crimes, argued that "economic sanctions are like a medieval siege but with a modern PR apparatus attached to justify what is being done." He went on to point out that "a difference is that such sieges used to be directed at starving out a single town or city while now they are aimed at squeezing whole countries into submission" (Cockburn 2018).

In the case of Syria, the United States and the European Union have implemented a growing range of sanctions. Since 1979, Washington has considered Syria a "state sponsor of terrorism." Since 2004, the export of US goods to Syria has been prevented. In 2011, this expanded to trade and import of Syrian oil. In addition, the United States has introduced "smart sanctions" against individuals from the Syrian government (Lund 2019).

The latest batch of US sanctions, known as the "Caesar Act," came into force in July 2020 (Caesar, 2020):

Under the Caesar Act, the US aims to hamper any foreign person who deals with the Damascus government, or the Iranian and Russian presence on the ground in support of the regime. They target sectors including construction, the military, and oil and gas, while the central bank could be labelled a "financial institution of primary money laundering concern." (Naharnet 2020)

The Caesar Act was named after the pseudonym of a Syrian intelligence dissident who leaked photo evidence of torture in Syria's intelligence branches. But the name also points, most likely unintentionally, to the use of the tactic of siege. In 52 BC the siege of Alesia was considered one of Julius Caesar's most successful military victories. As he recounted in his *Commentaries on the Gallic War*, Caesar decided to starve Alesia into surrendering through a brutal siege campaign: "When they came up to our fortifications, they wept and begged the soldiers to take them as slaves and give them something to eat. But I had guards posted all along the rampart with orders not to allow any of them inside our lines" (Livius 2001). It could therefore be considered an ominous signal that the United States decided in 2020 to name its sanctions against the Syrian government the Caesar Act.

Sanctions have been a weapon of choice for US administrations since the end of the Second World War. According to Gordon, two thirds of global sanctions from 1945 to the end of the 1990s were implemented by the United States—used to, among other things, secure trade objectives, enforce human rights, or generally ensure the maintenance of US hegemony (Gordon 1999a).

Although the Caesar Act is purportedly for the protection of civilians, it targets Syria's central bank as well as any financial transaction "that significantly facilitates the maintenance or expansion of the Government of Syria's domestic production of natural gas, petroleum, or petroleum products" or "knowingly, directly or indirectly, provides significant construction or engineering services to the Government of Syria." The sanctions are unashamedly intended to "deter foreign persons from entering into contracts related to reconstruction" (Caesar Act 2019).

This economic siege is intended to cripple Syria and force the surrender of, or political concessions from, those in positions of power. One condition outlined for the lifting of sanctions is that "areas besieged by the Government of Syria, the Government of the Russian Federation, the Government of Iran, or a foreign person described in section 102(a)(2)(A) (ii) are no longer cut off from international aid and have regular access to humanitarian assistance, freedom of travel, and medical care" (Caesar Act

2019). In short, the economic siege implemented by the United States will be lifted if the military siege implemented by the Syrian army is lifted.

In this way, the different types of siege imposed on Syrians come full circle. The siege against civilians in Syria triggers population movement, which triggers the reaction from neighboring states and Western governments to contain a population movement they fear, and which they try to control with border restrictions and punitive sanctions.

THE HUMAN COST

The human cost of these sieges is devastating. In Syria, areas under siege were decimated, with unimaginable consequences. Countless numbers of people were wounded or killed. Schools, mosques, markets, and health infrastructure were destroyed. Health services that did continue to function lacked supplies, leading to unnecessary suffering. Prices skyrocketed, leading to shortages of essential items. During the peak of the siege tactics, Médecins Sans Frontières/Doctors Without Borders (MSF) supported more than one hundred fifty medical facilities, focusing on besieged areas. In 2015, around Damascus alone, these facilities saw 93,162 war-wounded and recorded 4,634 war-dead. In areas under siege that same year, MSF documented forty-nine cases of death by starvation and sixty-three instances of medical facilities supported by MSF being shelled or bombed in airstrikes (MSF 2016b).

For Syrians in neighboring countries, the battle for survival did not involve bombs and bullets, but rather a policy-made misery, implemented to block people from reaching safety, entrap them in border zones, or force them back to Syria. If people managed to cross these borders, they encountered suffering on an enormous scale. For example, Shatila camp—originally for Palestinian refugees—mushroomed in size after the start of the war in Syria. What was once an overcrowded Palestinian camp has become an area where Syrian refugees, migrant workers, and Palestinian refugees—the most disenfranchised and neglected communities in Lebanon—live packed together in small spaces, one layer on top of another. Makeshift multistory buildings often have no running water or electricity. Because of the economic crisis, fuel is unaffordable for many people, and the camp in winter is cold, damp, and dark. In some homes people sleep in shifts due to the severe overcrowding.

In other parts of Lebanon, refugees live in informal tented settlements where they are exposed to the harsh winter elements. Those who have attempted to replace plastic sheeting with concrete walls have been forced to demolish them by Lebanese authorities who oppose the creation of formal camps (El Daoi 2020). Unsurprisingly, the poor living conditions for Syrian refugees have been a major determinant of poor health (Habib et al. 2019).

Refugees who have managed to make their way to Europe have encountered yet another policy-made assault on their lives and well-being. The capacity of the Greek island "hot spots" is estimated to be six thousand people. But the number of people crammed into these islands reached forty-two thousand in 2020. One in three of those refugees are children, many unaccompanied. The European Union policies resulting in the entrapment of this population have led to a major health crisis, particularly among children who are suffering severe mental health distress (Orcutt et al. 2020). In 2018, MSF teams reported

> multiple cases each week of teenagers who have attempted to commit suicide or self-harmed. Between February and June [2018], in a group mental health activity for children (aged between six and 18 years), MSF teams observed that nearly a quarter of the children participating (18 of 74 children) had self-harmed, attempted suicide or had thought about committing suicide. Other child patients were suffering from elective mutism, panic attacks, anxiety, aggressive outbursts and constant nightmares. (MSF 2018)

As for the sanctions imposed on Syria, Patrick Cockburn pointed out that "the record of economic sanctions in forcing political change is dismal, but as a way of reducing a country to poverty and misery it is difficult to beat" (Cockburn 2018). As with most sanctions regimes, in Syria there have been "humanitarian exemptions" to allow for the delivery of assistance into the country. But a leaked UN report from 2016 showed just how difficult it had been to implement these exemptions. "They cannot import the aid despite waivers because banks and commercial companies dare not risk being penalised for having anything to do with Syria. The report quotes a European doctor working in Syria as saying that 'the indirect effect of sanctions . . . makes the import of the medical instruments and other medical supplies immensely difficult, near impossible'" (Cockburn 2018).

By the middle of 2020, the sanctions on Syria already had contributed to an economic crisis, with the salary of a civil servant amounting to approximately US$20 per month (Parker 2020). With prices rising, food insecurity rose concurrently, not only among the eleven million people in need of humanitarian assistance as a result of the war, but also among those in areas relatively unaffected by the war (Parker 2020). According to a World Food Programme (WFP) survey in April 2020, a third of the Syrian population were not getting enough to eat, and 87 percent had no savings to help them through harder times (WFP 2020).

Idriss Jazairy, the UN rapporteur on sanctions, said that attempting to combat rights violations with sanctions was like trying "to extinguish a blaze with fire rather than water" (Lund 2019).

HUMANITARIAN COMPLICITY

Do the humanitarian implications of the sieges imposed on Syrians amount to a form of inhumane and degrading treatment, a collective punishment applied consistently by governments across the political spectrum? What is certain is that the application of the tactic of siege in Syria, in all its forms, has expanded together with the designation of civilian populations as enemies and terrorists. The humanitarian consequences have been devastating, and in many instances the humanitarian response has only reinforced the assault on Syrians' lives and dignity.

That the Syrian war has continued for so long, at such a brutal intensity and pace, is a major indictment of the post-World-War multilateral mechanisms of peace and security. Ultimately, Syria has been subjected to the impasse between two global powers, the United States and Russia, and two regional powers, Iran and Saudi Arabia. With no side willing or able to assert its full control over the situation, the people of Syria have been left to deal with the consequences of a protracted, bloody stalemate—one that has occurred in an era in which opposing forces have consensus on one thing: the expansive possibilities for attack offered by the war on terror.

The political paralysis representative of the war in Syria has been compounded by the humanitarian consequences of the tactics of warfare used by the belligerents. The delivery of humanitarian aid and the obstacles placed in the way of its distribution have become part of the battleground between warring factions. Each side in the Syrian war has controlled what it has deemed to be legitimate aid actions. From Damascus, the UN system and the International Committee of the Red Cross have struggled to deliver aid across front lines while respecting the desire of the Syrian government to appear in full control of the delivery of essential services to its citizens. In opposition-controlled areas, humanitarian organizations and activist networks have filled the gap left by the government and delivered aid considered by the Syrian state to be in direct violation of its sovereignty and an outright contestation of its legitimacy.[2] In neighboring countries and in Europe, humanitarian aid delivery, or its denial, has been used to orchestrate human misery as a deterrent to other migrants.

Ultimately, in these various forms of siege, humanitarian aid has been weaponized in the battle against an enemy broadly defined as criminals under the banner of both counterterrorism operations and the antimigration policies of right-wing nationalism (Munslow 2019).

Humanitarian aid has been offered in return for a political or military concession. In areas under military siege in Syria, humanitarian aid—including humanitarian ceasefires and corridors—often has been promised in return for a capitulation by the opposition on some specific term of negotiation or as part of a complete surrender. Along the closed borders surrounding Syria and in the policy of deterrence within neighboring countries, humanitarian aid has been denied, to ensure that conditions encourage people to return home to Syria. In Turkey, humanitarian aid offered by the European Union has gone a step further: Assistance is provided in exchange for Turkey agreeing to receive deported refugees and to prevent people from moving onward to Europe. In Europe itself, to deter new arrivals, camp conditions have been kept miserable and uninhabitable. Aid has been given to states that have agreed to act as the European Union's border guards.

To preserve the power of humanitarian aid as a weapon in the mechanisms of siege, it must be fully controlled by the besieging power. Aid actors that have operated outside the state's accepted parameters have been criminalized and come under attack in various forms from Syria to the shores of Europe (Whittall 2018).

In Syria, hospitals have been bombed and aid convoys attacked. In the border zones around Syria, humanitarian aid has been blocked, for example, from reaching refugees in "the Berm" between Jordan and Syria. Or humanitarians have been actively targeted and accused of supporting the enemy, as in the case of Turkey, where a number of humanitarian organizations have been expelled (Dettmer 2017). In Europe, search-and-rescue providers on the Mediterranean have been criminalized (Heller and Pezzani 2017).

In the Syrian war, humanitarian concerns have been a topic all sides and their backers could talk about and contest in place of having to meaningfully discuss the political roots of the war and its implementation through seige. Countless peace processes and UN Security Council deliberations have been dominated by disagreements over the delivery of humanitarian aid. A focus on Syrians' suffering has become the way in which seemingly intractable political negotiations have been ignored.

The UN Under-Secretary-General for Humanitarian Affairs and Emergency Relief Coordinator summed up the problem in his address to the press following a briefing of the Security Council in June 2016: "Besiegement is not a natural or necessary consequence of conflict, it is a deliberate policy of parties, and one which can be undone if the political will to do so can be mustered. While we work for more access, we have to keep in mind the only sustainable solution: a complete lifting of all sieges" (OCHA 2016). Siege Watch went further and spoke of the "futility, and irresponsibility, of substituting aid for political action" (Szybala et al. 2019, 28–29). Complicity of humanitarian actors can therefore also be seen in the way in which humanitarian concerns diverted attention away from the political choices to destroy peoples means of survival, in Syria and beyond, and the negotiated political agreements needed to end the crisis.

BREAKING THE CHAIN OF COMPLICITY

By examining siege from the perspective of the besieged, it becomes obvious that "the siege" does not end at the besieged city's borders. When a civilian manages to flee a siege, it follows them. This raises the question: Who are the ones truly being besieged? Is it the combatants, as claimed in the political discourse of the besiegers and implied in the basic definition of besiegement, or is it the population—unable to surrender—who have found themselves on the wrong side of an invisible front line in an ever expanding "with us or against us" war on terrorism in modern conflicts?

The case study of Syria shows that broadening the notion of siege gives a better sense of its real effects. The impact is almost always broader than the stated objective.

By broadening the notion of the siege we also gain better insight into the various actors involved. In Syria, siege-making goes beyond the obvious actors of Syria and Russia. The actors involved stretch from the warring parties themselves, to neighboring countries and populations pitted against refugees, to regional and global powers. The economic measures put in place to penalize the Syrian government—through sanctions—are ostensibly used as a punishment for sieges on Syrian cities, but in reality ensure the besiegement of the Syrian people.

Besieging combatants is a lawful act. Starving civilians and denying them assistance or the ability to seek refuge is not. As seen in each type of siege outlined above, this legal prohibition is circumvented by designating Syrians as terrorists—a label they are unable to shake off from cities under siege in Syria to the shores of Europe.

The rhetoric of those responsible for siege creates a smokescreen to hide unjustifiable policies. The Syrian government and its allies are fighting "terrorists." The US-led coalition does the same while claiming to be against the "regime," while Russia does the same while claiming to support the "sovereign state." Syria's neighbors are "destabilized," and Europe seeks to close its borders for "national security" purposes. Refugees are referred to as a "burden"—void of context and history—that needs to be shared, while the far right proclaims the security risks posed by "criminals" on the move.

All this rhetoric conveniently omits a set of fundamental facts. States have the responsibility to provide refuge to those fleeing war. There is also a responsibility to allow essential aid to reach those who need it, and to ensure that humanitarian aid is provided based on need instead of as a bargaining chip for political and military purposes. Instead, for Syrians, humanitarian suffering is caused by a political choice to destroy people's means of survival. The negotiations that ensued to ease this suffering were seldom about lifting the siege, but rather about allowing or disallowing humanitarian actors to mitigate against its worst effects.

It is only logical, and fair to the besieged, that we expand what we consider to be an act of besiegement to keep pace with the ways in which states have expanded whom they consider to be "terrorists." When entire communities can be considered terrorists—regardless of their physical location, affiliation, or intention—then so too can their experience of besiegement be considered continuous. The chain of complicity in Syrian suffering must be challenged and exposed, from the "anti-imperialist" Syrian government and its allies, to the "human rights"-promoting European Union and United States of America.

ACKNOWLEDGMENTS

I would like to thank Neve Gordon, Barry Munslow, Michiel Hofman, and Aurelie Ponthieu for their invaluable comments and input on earlier versions of this chapter.

NOTES

1. See Chapter 4 of this volume by Dawn Chatty.
2. See Chapter 7 of this volume by Alexey Khlebnikov.

REFERENCES

Adleh, Fadi, and Agnes Favier. 2017. "'Local Reconciliation Agreements' in Syria: A Non Starter for Peacebuilding." Middle East Directions. https://cadmus.eui.eu/bitstream/handle/1814/46864/RSCAS_MED_RR_2017_01.pdf?sequence=1.

Akkerman, Mark. 2018. "Expanding the Fortress: The Policies, the Profiteers, and the People Shaped by EU's Border Externalisation Programme." Transnational Institute. https://www.tni.org/en/publication/expanding-the-fortress.

Aldassouky, Ayman, and Sinan Hatahet. 2020. "The Role of Philanthropy in the Syrian War: Regime-Sponsored NGOs and Armed Group Charities." Middle East Directions. https://cadmus.eui.eu/bitstream/handle/1814/67370/RSCAS_RPR_2020_09.pdf?sequence=1&isAllowed=y.

Amnesty International. 2017. "We Leave or We Die: Forced Displacement under Syria's 'Reconciliation' Agreements." Amnesty International. https://www.amnesty.org/download/Documents/MDE2473092017ENGLISH.pdf.

BBC. 2020. "EU Chief Says Greece is Europe's Shield in Migrant Crisis." https://www.bbc.com/news/world-europe-51721356.

Beehner, Lionel M., Benedetta Berti, and Michael T. Jackson. 2017. "The Strategic Logic of Sieges in Counterinsurgencies." Parameters 47 (2). https://publications.armywarcollege.edu/pubs/3368.pdf.

Black, Ian. 2016. "Jordan Seals Borders After Suicide Attack." Guardian. https://www.theguardian.com/world/2016/jun/21/jordanian-soldiers-killed-by-car-bomb-outside-syrian-refugee-camp.

Bouchet-Saulnier, Françoise, and Jonathan Whittall. 2018. "An Environment Conducive to Mistakes? Lessons Learnt from the Attack on the Médecins Sans Frontières Hospital in Kunduz, Afghanistan." International Review of the Red Cross. https://international-review.icrc.org/articles/environment-conducive-mistakes-lessons-learnt-attack-medecins-sans-frontieres-hospital.

Caesar, 2020. (Syria Civilian Protection Act of 2019) H.R. 31, 116th Cong. (2019–2020). https://www.state.gov/caesar-syria-civilian-protection-act/

Chehayeb, Kareem. 2019. "Anti-Syrian Refugee Sentiment Ramps Up in Increasingly Hostile Lebanon." Middle East Eye. https://www.middleeasteye.net/news/anti-syrian-refugee-sentiment-ramps-increasingly-unwelcome-lebanon.

Cockburn, Patrick. 2018. "It's Time We Saw Economic Sanctions for What They Really Are—War Crimes." Independent. https://www.independent.co.uk/voices/economic-sanctions-north-korea-syria-hospital-supplies-a8168321.html.

Dettmer, Jamie. 2017. "Aid Groups Fear Mass Expulsion of Western NGOs from Turkey." Voice of America. https://www.voanews.com/europe/aid-groups-fear-mass-expulsion-western-ngos-turkey.

El Daoi, Racha. 2020. "Surviving Winter in a Tented Settlement." Norwegian Refugee Council. https://www.nrc.no/perspectives/2020/surviving-winter-in-a-tented-settlement/.

Fox, Major Amos C. 2018. "The Reemergence of the Siege: An Assessment of Trends in Modern Land Warfare." Association of the United States Army, Institute of Land Warfare. https://www.ausa.org/sites/default/files/LPE-18-2-The-Reemergence-of-the-Siege-An-Assessment-of-Trends-in-Modern-Land-Warfare.pdf.

Gordon, Joy. 1999a. "Economic Sanctions, Just War Doctrine, and the 'Fearful Spectacle of the Civilian Dead.'" CrossCurrents 49 (3), 387–400. https://www.jstor.org/stable/24460472?seq=1.

Gordon, Joy. 1999b. "Sanctions as Siege Warfare." Nation. March 4, 1999. https://www.thenation.com/article/archive/sanctions-siege-warfare/.

Gregory, Derek. 2011. "The Everywhere War." Geography Journal 177 (3), 238–250.

Rima R. Habib, Micheline Ziadee, Elio Abi Younes, Khalil El Asmar, and Mohammed Jawad. 2019. "The Association Between Living Conditions and Health Among

Syrian Refugee Children in Informal Tented Settlements in Lebanon." *Journal of Public Health* 42 (3), 323–333. doi:10.1093/pubmed/fdz108.

Hajjar, Lisa. 2016. "Israel as Innovator in the Mainstreaming of Extreme Violence." *Middle East Research and Information Project* (MERIP) 279 (Summer 2016). https://merip.org/2016/09/israel-as-innovator-in-the-mainstreaming-of-extreme-violence/

Hajjar, Lisa. 2019. "The Counterterrorism War Paradigm Versus International Humanitarian Law: The Legal Contradictions and Global Consequences of the US 'War on Terror.'" *Law & Social Inquiry* 44 (4), 922–956. doi:10.1017/lsi.2018.26.

Heller, Charles, and Lorenzo Pezzani. 2017. "Blaming the Rescuers." Forensic Oceanography. https://blamingtherescuers.org/.

HRW (Human Rights Watch). 2014. "Lebanon: At Least 45 Local Curfews Imposed on Syrian Refugees." HRW. https://www.hrw.org/news/2014/10/03/lebanon-least-45-local-curfews-imposed-syrian-refugees.

HRW (Human Rights Watch). 2017. "Lebanon: New Refugee Policy a Step Forward." HRW. https://www.hrw.org/news/2017/02/14/lebanon-new-refugee-policy-step-forward.

HRW (Human Rights Watch). 2018. "Turkey/Syria: Border Guards Shoot, Block Fleeing Syrians." HRW. https://www.hrw.org/news/2018/02/03/turkey/syria-border-guards-shoot-block-fleeing-syrians.

Hajžmanová, Ivana. 2017. "Syrians at the Berm: Surviving in Nightmarish Conditions and with an Uncertain Status." Internal Displacement Monitoring Centre. https://www.internal-displacement.org/expert-opinion/syrians-at-the-berm-surviving-in-nightmarish-conditions-and-with-an-uncertain-status.

Jackson, Michael, Lionel Beehner, and Benedetta Berti. 2016. "Modern Siege Warfare: How It Is Changing Counterinsurgency." *Foreign Affairs*. Date of publication 8 December, https://www.foreignaffairs.com/articles/syria/2016-12-07/modern-siege-warfare.

Janmyr, Maja. 2016. "Precarity in Exile: The Legal Status of Syrian Refugees in Lebanon." *Refugee Survey Quarterly* 35 (4), 58–78. https://academic.oup.com/rsq/article/35/4/58/2609281.

Livius. 2001. "Caesar on the Siege of Alesia." Last modified December 4, 2015. https://www.livius.org/sources/content/caesar/caesar-on-the-siege-of-alesia/.

Lund, Aron. 2019. "Briefing: Just How 'Smart' Are Sanctions on Syria?" *New Humanitarian*. https://www.thenewhumanitarian.org/analysis/2019/04/25/briefing-just-how-smart-are-sanctions-syria.

Monella, Lillo Montalto, and Sandrine Amiel. 2019. "Salvini Claims He Is Saving Europe from Islam, What Are the Facts?" Euronews. https://www.euronews.com/2019/05/03/europe-will-become-an-islamic-caliphate-if-we-don-t-take-back-control-salvini-tells-hunga.

MSF (Médecins Sans Frontières). 2016a. "Obstacle Course to Europe: A Policy Made Humanitarian Crisis at EU Borders." https://www.msf.org/sites/msf.org/files/msf_obstacle_course_to_europe_0.pdf.

MSF (Médecins Sans Frontières). 2016b. "Syria 2015: "Documenting war-wounded and war -dead in MSF-supported medical facilities in Syria". https://www.msf.org/sites/msf.org/files/2018-05/syria_2015_war-dead_and_war-wounded_report_en.pdf.

MSF (Médecins Sans Frontières). 2018. "Increasing Suicide Attempts and Self-Harming Among Child Refugees Trapped in Moria Camp, Lesvos." News release. https://prezly.msf.org.uk/increasing-suicide-attempts-and-self-harming-among-child-refugees-trapped-in-moria-camp-lesvos.

Munslow, Barry. 2019. "Humanitarianism Under Attack." *International Health* 11 (5), 358–360. https://doi.org/10.1093/inthealth/ihz065.

Naharnet Newsdesk. 2020. "How Will New U.S. Sanctions Impact Syria and Lebanon?" Naharnet. http://www.naharnet.com/stories/en/272603-how-will-new-u-s-sanctions-impact-syria-and-lebanon.

OCHA (UN Office for the Coordination of Humanitarian Affairs). 2016. "Under-Secretary-General for Humanitarian Affairs and Emergency Relief Coordinator, Stephen O'Brien Security Council Briefing on Humanitarian Access in Syria." News release. https://reliefweb.int/report/syrian-arab-republic/under-secretary-general-humanitarian-affairs-and-emergency-relief-40.

OHCHR (Office of the United Nations High Commissioner for Human Rights). 2018. "Abuse Behind Bars: Arbitrary and Unlawful Detention in Libya." OHCHR. https://www.ohchr.org/Documents/Countries/LY/AbuseBehindBarsArbitrary Unlawful_EN.pdf.

Orcutt, Miriam, Reem Mussa, Lucinda Hiam, Apostolos Veizis, Sophie McCann, Elisavet Papadimitriou, Aurelie Ponthieu, and Michael Knipper. 2020. "EU Migration Policies Drive Health Crisis on Greek Islands." *Lancet.* https://www.thelancet.com/journals/lancet/article/PIIS0140-6736(19)33175-7/fulltext.

Parker, Ben. 2020. "Inflation, Shortages Worsen Syrian Poverty on Eve of New US Sanctions." *New Humanitarian.* https://www.thenewhumanitarian.org/news/2020/06/09/Syria-economic-crisis-currency-exchange-rate-crash-us-sanctions.

Perugini, Nicola, and Neve Gordon. 2018. "The Global War on Migration, Human Shields, and the Erosion of the Civilian." *Humanity Journal* (blog). http://humanityjournal.org/blog/perugini-and-gordon/.

Ponthieu, Aurelie. 2015. "Words of Concern, Walls of Deterrence: Refugees Pushed Out to Sea." MSF-Analysis. https://msf-analysis.org/words-of-concern-walls-of-deterrence-refugees-pushed-out-to-sea/

Ponthieu, Aurelie. 2016. "Why the EU's Deal with Turkey Is No Solution to the 'Crisis' Affecting Europe." MSF. https://www.msf.org/migration-why-eu%E2%80%99s-deal-turkey-no-solution-%E2%80%9Ccrisis%E2%80%9D-affecting-europe.

Saghieh, Nizar. 2015. "Manufacturing Vulnerability in Lebanon: Legal Policies as Efficient Tools of Discrimination." *Legal Agenda.* https://www.legal-agenda.com/en/article.php?id=3068.

Schultheis, Emily. 2019. "How the Far Right Weaponized Europe's Interior Ministries to Block Refugees." *Atlantic.* https://www.theatlantic.com/international/archive/2019/03/europe-interior-minister-kickl-far-right/584845/.

Sidahmed, Asil. 2017. "De-Escalation Zones in Syria—Not an Alternative for Refugees." MSF Analysis. https://msf-analysis.org/de-escalation-zones-syria-not-alternative-refugees/.

SNHR (Syrian Network for Human Rights). 2017. "The Syrian Regime Has Dropped Nearly 70,000 Barrel Bombs on Syria." SNHR. https://reliefweb.int/sites/reliefweb.int/files/resources/The_Syrian_Regime_Has_Dropped_Nearly_70%2C000_Barrel_Bombs_en.pdf.

Sparrow, Annie. 2018. "How UN Humanitarian Aid Has Propped Up Assad." *Foreign Affairs.* Date of publication 22 September, https://www.foreignaffairs.com/articles/syria/2018-09-20/how-un-humanitarian-aid-has-propped-assad.

Syrian Observatory for Human Rights. 2020. "Syrian Revolution Nine Years On: 586,100 Persons Killed and Millions of Syrians Displaced and Injured." https://www.syriahr.com/en/157193/.

Szybala, Valerie and the Team. 2019. "Siege Watch, Final Report—Out of Sight, Out of Mind: The Aftermath of Syria's Sieges." PAX. https://reliefweb.int/sites/reliefweb.int/files/resources/pax-siege-watch-final-report.pdf.

Terre des Hommes Foundation, Save the Children, and World Vision. 2019. "Demolition of Syrian Homes in Arsal: At Least 15,000 Children Will Be Made Homeless." News release. https://www.tdh.ch/en/press-releases/demolition-syrian-homes-arsal-least-15000-children-will-be-made-homeless.

Todman, Will. 2017. "The Resurgence of Siege Warfare." *CCAS Newsmagazine*. https://issuu.com/georgetownsfs/docs/ccasnewsfw2017_final_issuu.

United Nations General Assembly (UNGA)—Human Rights Council. 2017. "Report of the Independent International Commission of Inquiry on the Syrian Arab Republic." https://undocs.org/A/HRC/34/64

UNHCR (Office of the United Nations High Commissioner for Refugees). 2020a. "Lebanon: Protection." UNHCR. https://www.unhcr.org/lb/protection.

UNHCR (Office of the United Nations High Commissioner for Refugees). 2020b. "Syria Emergency." UNHCR. https://www.unhcr.org/syria-emergency.html.

Urban Operations. 2006. Headquarters, Department of the Army. https://fas.org/irp/doddir/army/fm3-06.pdf.

Van Schaack, Beth. 2016. "Siege Warfare and the Starvation of Civilians as a Weapon of War and War Crime." Just Security. https://www.justsecurity.org/29157/siege-warfare-starvation-civilians-war-crime/.

Vohra, Anchal. 2019a. "Lebanon Is Sick and Tired of Syrian Refugees." *Foreign Policy*. https://foreignpolicy.com/2019/07/31/lebanon-is-sick-and-tired-of-syrian-refugees/.

Vohra, Anchal. 2019b. "Lebanon, Turkey Act Against Syrian Refugees." Observer Research Foundation. https://www.orfonline.org/expert-speak/lebanon-turkey-act-against-syrian-refugees-54035/.

Walt, Vivienne. 2019. "Hungary's Far-Right Government Has Been Getting a Boost from President Trump Ahead of E.U. Elections." *Time*. Date of publication 22 May. https://time.com/5590134/hungary-foreign-minister-interview/.

WFP (World Food Programme). 2020. "Syria m-VAM" Bulletin. https://docs.wfp.org/api/documents/WFP-0000115728/download/?iframe.

Whittall, Jonathan. 2016. "Treating Terrorists." *Jadaliyya*. https://www.jadaliyya.com/Details/33495.

Whittall, Jonathan. 2018. "The Politics of Health in Counterterrorism Operations." *Middle East Report* 286. https://merip.org/2018/10/the-politics-of-health-in-counterterrorism-operations/.

Zerofsky, Elisabeth. 2019. "Viktor Orbán's Far-Right Vision for Europe." *New Yorker*. Date of Publication 7 January, https://www.newyorker.com/magazine/2019/01/14/viktor-orbans-far-right-vision-for-europe.

CHAPTER 7

Information Warfare and the Role of Global Humanitarians

ALEXEY KHLEBNIKOV

Since the dawn of the modern era of international aid, humanitarian organizations have been accused of creating and spreading distorted facts, images, and disinformation about parties to conflicts or the conflicts themselves. At the same time, humanitarians present on the ground have become essential subactors and even full-scale nonstate actors in almost every conflict—although the degree and scale of their presence may vary. And because international humanitarian organizations represent specific values, interests, and demands that go beyond state borders, this makes them pivotal actors on the global stage—actors with the power to influence conflict dynamics by contributing to the worldwide dissemination and translation of certain narratives and images. Such power can be used in a destructive and manipulative way that contributes to the spread of biased information and narratives, which can have a serious impact on a conflict's evolution.

To understand the mechanisms and problems of the narratives created and produced by humanitarians, it helps to review the history of contemporary humanitarian organizations' formation, as well as their role and the activities they have participated in over time.

Institutional humanitarianism is in essence a product of European civilization and Western liberal thought. With the extension of citizens' rights in Europe and North America in the nineteenth century, people began establishing independent associations, organizations,[1] and labor

Alexey Khlebnikov, *Information Warfare and the Role of Global Humanitarians* In: *Everybody's War.* Edited by: Jehan Bseiso, Michiel Hofman, and Jonathan Whittall, Oxford University Press. © Médecins Sans Frontières 2021.
DOI: 10.1093/oso/9780197514641.003.0008

unions that served as instruments for meeting community or professional needs, defending their interests, or promoting new policies. These were the first nongovernmental organizations (NGOs)—which over the following decades, and through the First and the Second World Wars, would grow and extend their reach internationally, all the while spreading their interests and ideas. During the Cold War period, many humanitarian agencies formed part of some countries' so-called soft power (such as the United States, United Kingdom, Federal Republic of Germany, and France), helping to promote positive images of these countries, their ideologies, and their values alongside the organizations' humanitarian assistance.

The end of the Cold War, which ushered in a Western liberal-democratic paradigm that dominated for almost two decades, not only changed the globe politically and economically, but also had an impact on humanitarian assistance and organizations. A shift toward democratization combined with technological advances (via the information revolution) created the perfect conditions for civil society groups and NGOs to thrive. The end of the Cold War also led to the domination of a liberal humanitarian peace-building agenda, which provided many NGOs with more space and tools to promote that particular cause.

In addition, the end of the Cold War created a new normative environment, initiating numerous regional conflicts and new threats. Within this environment, international NGOs (INGOs) found more space in which to operate (Stephenson and Zanotti 2012), in many ways thanks to a change in the way Western leaders started to think about and respond to fresh challenges (McMahon 2017). Western states now began delegating humanitarian activities in conflicts to INGOs, which they viewed as more flexible and cost-efficient.

Since 1990, the number of INGOs has grown rapidly. In the 1950s there were about one thousand; in the 1980s about four thousand; and in the 1990s about six thousand. That number increased to twenty-six thousand in 1999, and to forty thousand in 2013 (Ben-Ari 2013). In other words, the number of INGOs boomed after the end of the Cold War and the so-called end of history, when the Western liberal-capitalist paradigm won over the Soviet-socialist one.

Also starting in the 1990s, the Western military approach to conflicts worldwide was frequently framed in terms of the new concept of "humanitarian intervention," which allowed nations to justify or explain military involvement through the lens of respect for human rights and humanitarian assistance to the civilian population (Robinson 2002). Part of this concept was codified in the Responsibility to Protect (R2P) doctrine adopted by the United Nations General Assembly in 2005 (UNGA 2005 par. 138, 139). As a result, humanitarian interventions have been built into Western military doctrine, justified on humanitarian grounds, often as part of a strategy to "win hearts and minds." Michael Barnett, a US scholar who focuses on humanitarian issues in politics, has argued that such approaches and policies have had a serious impact on the behavior of humanitarian NGOs and have often co-opted them, resulting at times in humanitarians capturing and disseminating propaganda (Barnett 2005).

In general, the global political landscape has changed rapidly in the first two decades of the new millennium and with it the operational environment for humanitarian organizations. Many INGOs seem to have struggled to adapt to this new reality. "The end of history" did not happen, and a unipolar, Western-dominated world order failed to crystalize its supremacy. Instead, the West's attempts at global domination have failed, and may even have contributed to a host of new challenges and complications: increased polarization around the world (West versus East, North versus South); the rise of new power centers (Brazil, Russia, India, China, South Africa—"BRICS"); a resurgence of regionalization and development of regional organizations— for example, the Shanghai Cooperation Organization (SCO), the Eurasian Economic Union, the Russia-led Collective Security Treaty Organization (CSTO), BRICS bank, the Asian Infrastructure Investment Bank (AIIB), and the Association of Southeast Asian Nations (ASEAN); the undermining and erosion of global institutions and international treaties—including the United Nations, the Organization for Security and Co-operation in Europe (OSCE), the Arab League, the World Trade Organization, and the Intermediate-Range Nuclear Forces (INF) treaty; the rise of radicalism in and uncontrolled migration flows from the Middle East and North Africa; and reinvigorated sovereignty and nationalism around the world.

Despite these developments, the majority of INGOs are still Western-born and -located, which has affected their approaches and behavior. About 70 percent of all INGOs are located in the West (Zonova 2013). About 30 percent of the 5,451 INGOs that have consultative status[2] in the United Nations (UN) are located in the United States (the Borgen Project 2016). At the same time, the majority of INGO activities are conducted in Africa, the Middle East, and Asia—all different and rapidly changing environments. In this context, one of the main challenges for humanitarian INGOs is to adapt to a changing world order so different from the one in which they emerged. Yet the majority of today's INGOs are trying to fit their old, traditional systems and approaches into these altered contexts, rather than adapting (Start Network 2013). The rise of a polycentric world order in which humanitarians have struggled to change or update their thinking and practices has contributed to the instrumentalization of aid actors by warring parties. This often has occurred through some INGOs participating in creating political and military narratives—that is, propaganda.

HUMANITARIAN INTERNATIONAL NONGOVERNMENTAL ORGANIZATIONS AS GLOBAL ACTORS

In the context of military conflict with an intensifying "information warfare" component, the role of humanitarian organizations also has been transformed. In many ways INGOs have become sovereign actors of global politics, able to act on their own and even to undermine the sovereignty of a state when they operate across borders without its consent. At the same time, INGOs in many contexts remain instrumental to certain states' and other entities' interests and approaches to conflict. Acknowledging the tension between state sovereignty and INGOs' capacity to act independently seems central to understanding other issues connected to humanitarian INGOs' activities in conflict zones.

Humanitarian INGOs represent certain values (e.g., human rights, democracy), advocate particular interests (e.g., push for cross-border aid deliveries in Syria, boycotting working with Damascus), make demands and enforce policies (e.g., call for free and transparent aid flow and distribution, advocate for regime change, demand justice for [war] crimes), and operate with substantial human and financial resources (in 2017 humanitarian NGOs spent $16.6 billion; [Knox Clarke 2018]). Moreover, INGOs initiate, contribute to, and participate in many international initiatives and actions, which has brought them recognition as nonstate actors in the world political system (Paul 2000; Lebedeva and Kharkevich 2013). Humanitarian INGOs often influence global politics—sometimes in a way that can negatively affect the interests of individual states. In this way, INGOs' sovereignty of action intersects with state sovereignty, which can lead to a violation of the latter.

This clash of sovereignty is particularly pronounced in Syria, where the majority of humanitarian INGOs have worked cross-border throughout the conflict. Based in Turkey, Jordan, and Iraq (with the consent of each of the hosting states), humanitarians have run their operations in Syria in territories outside the Syrian government's control. The Syrian government, in turn, has viewed these activities as illegal and as undermining its sovereignty, because the INGOs have operated without its consent. In the government's eyes, the INGOs have aided terrorists, which the government has regarded as legitimate grounds to deny these INGOs the ability to conduct their operations legally, through Damascus.

One could contend that the Syrian government has reason to be suspicious of the INGOs' motives, because a high number of INGOs are concentrated in the West and are primarily funded by the Western states, which influences their approach toward the Syrian authorities. As a result, Damascus views Western INGOs as agents of Western states' interests, which conflicts with the interests of the Syrian government.

One could argue that more INGOs are founded in the West because they usually appear in liberal environments and democracies, rather than in authoritarian regimes, where it is harder, if not impossible, to start and run an NGO. One could also argue, however, that because the West is the most economically developed and prosperous part of the world, INGOs based there can more easily raise the necessary funds for their operational activities. This fundraising aspect alone poses a problem: The majority of INGO funding still comes from the West, and often directly from Western governments—a situation that creates an original bias in the INGOs' policies and activities.

For example, in the 1990s, the UN High Commissioner for Refugees (UNHCR) expressed alarm that governments were increasingly channeling funds for humanitarian assistance to their own national NGOs, rather than to multilateral agencies like itself (Krieger 2001), which left the UNHCR less active due to the lack of funding. By the late 1990s, European Union (EU) funding directly to NGOs increased to about $1.5 billion from about $1 billion in the first half of the decade. At the end of the 1990s, government grants represented 40 percent of NGO budgets, compared with 1.5 percent in 1970 (Paul 2000). By 2017, money from Western governments and EU institutions made up 76 percent of total international humanitarian assistance (Knox Clarke 2018). This trend inevitably exposed humanitarian INGOs to increased pressure from donor governments; though it allowed them to grow their operational capabilities, it also limited their independence.

This development made humanitarian INGOs more exposed to being instrumentalized in their efforts to provide aid. According to a 2018 report by Active Learning Network for Accountability and Performance (ALNAP), a global network of NGOs, UN agencies, and other actors and experts in the humanitarian aid community, most institutional funding continued to come from a small group of government and multilateral donors—the largest twenty donors provided 96 percent of the institutional total in 2017. Contributions from the three largest government donors—the United States, Germany, and the United Kingdom—accounted for 56 to 59 percent of all government contributions in 2014–2017. Although the majority of government funding traditionally goes to UN agencies as first-level recipients (about 60 percent, or $12.3 billion, in 2016), UN agencies then further allocate funds to humanitarian NGOs as second-level recipients. In the end, the biggest UN funders have a say in how and where UN humanitarian funds are best used. In addition, 34 percent of government funding goes directly to NGOs.

It should be noted that some INGOs have decided not to accept funding from governments in conflict areas (Médecins Sans Frontières), or not to accept government funding at all (Greenpeace). Still, most humanitarian INGOs—which remain crucial providers of humanitarian assistance during times of conflict—depend heavily on governmental funding. Thus, states in conflict, such as Syria, tend to be suspicious toward INGOs working in their territory. The INGOs become seen as tools of foreign governments pursuing their own interests, and trying to undermine the sovereignty of the state in question.

The combination of humanitarian INGOs' global influence and their dependence on funding from Western states is why many states, who are party to a conflict, are often afraid of, and treat with suspicion, the presence of INGOs in their territory. This tension is especially pronounced in Syria, where many humanitarians have acted without the government's consent and have conducted cross-border operations. This problem of state sovereignty, how it is treated by other actors, and how to regulate relations between state and nonstate actors, or among nonstate actors, is an enormous challenge, and one that requires more attention.

CONCEPTUAL DISSONANCE AND UNEXPECTED IMPLICATIONS IN AID PROVISION

Despite humanitarians' noble mission and goals, their activities during conflicts may easily cause controversial results. This dissonance happens due to the nature of modern conflicts. Previously, colonial and interstate conflicts accounted for half of all armed conflicts, but these types of conflicts have all but disappeared. In 2017 only one conflict, in Kashmir, was a dispute between two countries: India and Pakistan. Today, the predominant form of conflict is intrastate (internal to a state), although it often involves external state actors (Dupuy and Rustad 2018). According to a study by the Peace Research Institute Oslo, such internationalized conflicts—civil wars with external parties involved—are more durable and less likely to find a political solution. This durability can be caused by the nature of the conflict itself but may also be driven by the increasing number of parties involved, which means more actors to potentially block a deal for resolution (Håvard,

Rustad, Urdal, Nygård 2019). The rise in prevalence of civil or intrastate conflicts has complicated the operational environment for INGOs, blurred distinctions between military and civilian actors, and increased the risk that INGOs will be seen as not neutral.

Additional factors on the ground complicate the work of humanitarian INGOs and increase their level of instrumentalization by parties to the conflict. The case of the Syrian war is even more complex because the armed opposition has been highly fragmented. This means that plenty of competing armed groups control different areas and different populations, fighting not only Syrian government forces but also one another. As a result, humanitarian agencies have had to work on the ground with a variety of often competing actors to gain access to targeted populations in need. Although humanitarian INGOs have the capacity and ability to work in both government and opposition-held areas in Syria, for the majority, their main operations have focused almost exclusively on areas outside Damascus's control. This situation often has put them between a rock and a hard place and has promoted a narrative pushed by Damascus that humanitarians are not genuinely neutral and have contributed to the prolongation of the conflict.

This assertion that humanitarians prolong conflict is not entirely without grounds. Research has shown several ways in which INGO activity can contribute to the endurance of a conflict or even lead to an increase in the rate of violence (Anderson 1996, 1999; Marsden 1997; Cooley and Ron 2002). First, humanitarian aid delivered to civilians in need can be appropriated by the parties to the conflict. This aid is a valuable resource for warring parties and can be easily commandeered to support fighting efforts, enhance capabilities, and maintain or increase resilience. During the Syrian conflict, humanitarian aid including medical material and food designated for civilians often has ended up in the hands of opposition fighters, including those designated as terrorist organizations by Syria or the United Nations, such as the Islamic State of Iraq and Sham (ISIS), Jabhat al-Nusra, Hayat Tahrir al-Sham, Jaysh al-Islam, and Faylaq al-Rahman. In the same manner, humanitarian aid provided by organizations that worked with the Syrian government often did not reach designated civilian populations and was instead distributed among soldiers or pro-government militias. The question arises whether humanitarians have the capacity to control distribution of aid effectively given the complex and insecure operational environment.

Second, warring parties can impose entrance fees or other taxation on humanitarians for the right to work and deliver aid to civilians. As a result, some of the resources designated for civilians are instead passed on to fighters. Suspicions of such taxation were numerous during the Syrian conflict,[3] which the Syrian government used to justify its negative position toward INGOs operating in the country.

Third, warring parties receive indirect benefits from the infrastructure built by humanitarian INGOs and intended for general benefit (e.g., roads, hospitals, power stations, water-pumping stations), which can enhance the positions of parties to the conflict. Some INGOs and Western governments use the following logic (Lund 2018; Darden 2019; Cambanis and Heller 2018) in describing their refusal to cooperate with Damascus: If we build new roads for Bashar al-Assad, he will use them to advance his military offensives and continue to oppress his own population; if we build hospitals for Assad, he will treat his soldiers there instead of civilians in need; power stations we reconstruct will be used by Assad to gain more public support. This logic—which reflects a view of the Syrian government as a nontransparent and unreliable partner—has only worsened the humanitarian situation in the country, as government-held areas host millions of people in need, including internally displaced persons (IDPs). In 2019, 7.2 million out of a total 11.7 million Syrians in need[4] lived in government-controlled areas, as did 3.8 million out of a total 6.2 million IDPs (Humanitarian Needs Overview 2019). As a result, an enormous number of Syrians in need and the displaced were out of reach of many humanitarian organizations. The situation in government-held areas is further complicated by international sanctions and the United States' 2019 Caesar Syria Civilian Protection Act,[5] which greatly obstructs the delivery of humanitarian aid to government-held areas.

Fourth, humanitarian aid can enhance the war economy. Such aid frees up resources intended for the civilian population under warring parties' control, resources that can then be diverted to the war effort, or at least to ease the financial burden of warring parties. This has applied to all sides of the conflict in Syria.[6]

Fifth, according to the British researcher Peter Marsden, humanitarian INGOs can directly contribute to war efforts (Marsden 1997). Marsden offers the example of Afghanistan in the 1980s, when humanitarian INGOs operated exclusively in mujahideen-held areas of the country. Almost the same has happened in Syria. And because medical humanitarian aid includes the obligation to provide medical care to wounded combatants, such care— of wounded mujahideen fighters then and Syrian fighters now—becomes a particularly sensitive issue if INGOs work only on one side. The US scholars Alexander Cooley and James Ron (2002) also highlight that humanitarian work in refugee camps may contribute to wider conflicts, providing the example of INGOs working in camps in Goma, Democratic Republic of the

Congo, in 1994–1995. NGOs working there were widely criticized because their humanitarian relief efforts were vastly compromised by the presence of Hutu fighters, who used the camps as safe havens and bases from which to launch attacks against civilians (MSF 2004).

In Syria, the majority of humanitarian agencies have worked exclusively in areas outside government control, which has contributed to the resilience of opposition fighters and to Kurdish groups' capacity to keep fighting. This occurred partly because the Syrian government did not allow many humanitarian INGOs to work in Syria officially, or created many obstacles to their operating in government-held areas; and partly because some INGOs did not want to work with the Syrian government. In addition, many opposition fighters, including the more radical ones, used refugee camps and the territories of other countries (Turkey, Jordan) as bases from which to fight Syrian government forces. There, they had access to humanitarian assistance and received support, not only from INGOs, but also directly from foreign states, and could use these territories as a safe haven. As a result, humanitarian assistance can be said to have contributed to the prolongation and intensity of the conflict.

Finally—and especially important—humanitarian INGOs can contribute to the extension of conflict by stoking adversarial attitudes within and between parties, increasing polarization and antagonism. Today, one of humanitarian INGOs' key activities is advocacy, which often involves collecting and publicizing human rights abuses and violations and disseminating this information globally. Although advocacy can at times have a positive impact in improving the conditions for civilians trapped in a war, it also can have unintended consequences, such as contributing to the polarization between the parties to a conflict, as INGOs have been increasingly implicated in "information warfare"—that is, in spreading propaganda. This can worsen the situation on the ground, contributing to the polarization between the parties to a conflict. It easily provokes defensive, or even offensive, responses and increased outrage from the perpetrators of violations, contributing to their dehumanization not only within their country, but also in the broader region and around the world. The spread of these narratives can alienate the parties further and undermine all attempts at reconciliation and the creation of a lasting political settlement. Moreover, it hardens parties' opposition to one another and fails to help decrease hostilities.

For example, the dominant narrative of the Syria war formed in the West is that the Syrian government is solely responsible for almost everything negative that has happened. But there are no saints in civil wars.

Undoubtedly, the Syrian government is responsible for many crimes, but so is the armed opposition, which includes many fighters designated as terrorist groups, not only by the Syrian state, but also by the UN and Western states. In absolute terms, the Syrian government bears more responsibility simply because its capacity to use power was initially much greater than that of the armed opposition. But at the same time, foreign sponsors and international support networks (Bellin 2004) provided the armed opposition with necessary resources and assistance, which allowed them to fight the Syrian Army, its affiliates, and civilians who remained loyal to the government, as well as other competing armed groups. Yet the dominant narrative remained one of violence almost exclusively committed by the Syrian state—a narrative that took hold partly due to the much higher presence of humanitarian INGOs in opposition-held areas compared with government-controlled regions, and partly due to INGO access to a wide set of digital communication tools, which enabled the rapid spread of messages and images from opposition areas. This one-sided narrative contributed heavily to the growing alienation and intransigence between the opposition and the government, making any meaningful dialogue between them nearly impossible.

Narratives are not formed in a vacuum. To ensure the smooth conduct of their operations, humanitarian INGOs make many decisions: They decide whom to hire (some people but not others), purchase goods and services from certain people (and not others), deliver aid to one group of people (but not to others). These decisions can create separate group identities, inequalities, and jealousies, which often contribute to polarization within communities (Anderson 1996). As a result, it can be argued that in situations such as Syria, humanitarian INGOs indirectly (and sometimes directly) influence the behavior of individuals and even certain communities and parties to the conflict who are directly involved in violence. As a result, humanitarian aid can contribute to increasing polarization between (or within) the parties of conflict. Undoubtedly, INGOs contribute far less to the violence than do the local armed groups directly involved in combat, the state, or international military forces. But it is important to underline that INGOs do play some role and should therefore take responsibility; their part in contributing to violence should be analyzed and, as much as possible, prevented. All INGOs, humanitarian or otherwise, working in sensitive conflict environments must thoroughly evaluate all possible consequences and impacts of their activities, whether on-the-ground delivery of humanitarian aid or online documenting and publicizing of human rights violations and crimes.

Let's look at some cases where various types of INGOs were implicated, intentionally or unintentionally, in information warfare, or propaganda—the creation and dissemination of certain narratives about parties to some conflicts.

In 2011, in Libya, Amnesty International (AI) contributed to the push for United Nations Security Council (UNSC) action, which eventually led to humanitarian intervention. It often promoted and reinforced claims of potential abuses of human rights by the Libyan government (Amnesty International 2011; Kovalik 2012; Taylor 2014), although it later disproved them. Interestingly, a report released in 2016 by the United Kingdom's House of Commons Foreign Affairs Select Committee found that in 2011 the UK government "failed to identify that the threat to civilians was overstated and that the rebels included a significant Islamist element," and that widespread concerns prior to the R2P intervention in Libya regarding "the scale of threat to civilians was presented with unjustified certainty" (House of Commons Foreign Affairs Committee 2016). Judging by this report, it appears that AI misrepresented events in Libya, which contributed to the construction and promotion of the then dominant regime-change narrative.

This appears to repeat itself in Syria. AI has also heavily influenced public perceptions about the Syrian conflict, pushing the narrative that the Assad-led Syrian government has been the party primarily responsible for war crimes and crimes against humanity (Amnesty International 2012). Tim Hayward, a professor at the University of Edinburgh, has analyzed the evidence AI has used to back some of its claims and found that it has not always stuck to its own protocols while conducting its analyses. Hence, some of AI's claims appear unsupported, which contributes to the argument that it has presented a biased picture of the conflict (Hayward 2017).

A significant controversy also was caused by the White Helmets organization in Syria (also known as the Syria Civil Defense), which presented itself as an independent NGO set up to save civilians. Critics, however, point out that this independent NGO received its major funds from the United States Agency for International Development (USAID; Craddick 2017), both directly[7] and indirectly through the for-profit development firm Chemonics International, and from the UK government.[8] Critics also argue that the group's main goal is dissemination of propaganda designed to promote a "regime-change" narrative (Morningstar 2014). The White Helmets operate near or within the territories of opposition groups, including those affiliated with Jabhat al-Nusra, Hayat Tahrir al-Sham, Ahrar al-Sham, and Nur al-Din al-Zinki (Beeley 2015a).[9] Observers have reported that workers and volunteers with the NGO have been seen in pro-radical group demonstrations and even during fighting, filming executions (Beeley 2015b).[10] Supporters of the group said that the White Helmets contributed to "an invaluable reporting and advocacy role" and supported "confidence to statements made by UK and other international leaders made in condemnation of Russian actions" (Mason 2017). The NGO also serves as the "most routinely used reliable source of reporting" for organizations such as Human Rights Watch (HRW) and AI.[11] Most major Western media, in turn, often (if not always) take information from reports by HRW and AI as well as from opposition forces (Simons 2019, 443–60). But because the White Helmets operate exclusively in opposition-held areas, where they can draw only a partial picture of events (events that are difficult to independently verify), this contributes to the creation and spread of a one-sided narrative about the Syrian conflict. Thus, the informational part of the organization's activities looks—intentionally or not—increasingly propagandistic.

This bias is further enhanced by the White Helmets' positioning of themselves as an exclusive Syrian first-response medical humanitarian organization helping victims of the conflict, using the secondary name Syria Civil Defense (السوري الدفاع المدني). Another organization with a similar name—the Syrian Civil Defense Forces[12]—has been active in Syria since 1953, long before the White Helmets were created. To reach out to the official Syrian Civil Defense Forces, you call 113 inside Syria. This is a certified Syrian civil defense and rescue organization, a part of the country's defense system and member of the International Civil Defense Organization (ICDO) since 1972. ICDO has an observer status with UN General Assembly[13] and has cooperation agreements signed with the World Health Organization (WHO) and the International Committee of the Red Cross (ICRC).[14] Its main task is to protect and assist the civilian population in times of conflict or natural disaster, and to participate in the reconstruction of damaged infrastructure. During the recent conflict, the Syria Civil Defense Forces operated in both government- and opposition-held areas up to 2016, when it ceased to work in opposition-held areas due to security reasons, after the opposition had deliberately targeted its crew members during rescue missions. Thereafter, the Syria Civil Defense Forces continued to serve at least 60 percent of the Syrian population under government control, including million IDPs.

Yet the White Helmets—echoing the name of an existing Syrian organization and using it in their media communications—successfully created a narrative implying they were the sole authentic Syrian civil defense organization acting at the epicenter of the conflict. The handful of reports about the original Syria Civil Defense Forces went mostly unnoticed by Western audiences.

Among humanitarian INGOs, the well-known and widely respected Médecins Sans Frontières (MSF) is one of many that has faced huge challenges during the Syrian conflict. Its reports are at constant risk of being manipulated by the media, and thus it has inadvertently contributed to the formation of a distorted picture of the Syria war. MSF's programs in Syria have operated almost exclusively in areas outside government control (notwithstanding many negotiations to start operations in government areas), which has negatively affected its image as a neutral actor. In addition, media sympathetic to different parties to the conflict have been quick to use MSF communications for their own purposes: Opposition supporters have praised MSF's work, while Syrian government supporters have criticized MSF as being one-sided, for sometimes helping so-called terrorists and for contributing to the dissemination of propaganda.

Moreover, since 2014, MSF international staff members have not been constantly on the ground in opposition-held areas, although the organization has maintained an international presence in Kurdish-controlled areas. Before 2014, MSF had international staff on the ground to run its projects in most areas. But with time it became harder for the organization to negotiate with armed groups regarding the territories where they could work. At the start of 2014, ISIS abducted five of MSF's colleagues, which forced the group to pull international staff out of Syria for security reasons.[15] Therefore, in these opposition-held areas, MSF no longer has access to external sources to verify information; it now must rely, as do many other NGOs, exclusively on its local networks. In many cases, information on the ground has come from people working in areas under the control of more radical armed groups, including designated terrorist groups (such as ISIS or Jabhat al-Nusra/Hayat Tahrir al-Sham), which raises the question of whether the information received has been shared only with their permission and under their protection. This, in turn, raises the question of how reliable such uncorroborated information is—that is, whether it has come from potentially compromised sources.

Yet after the departure of most of its international staff, MSF repeatedly released statements (MSF 2016, 2020; Shaheen 2016) in which it assigned responsibility for airstrikes on hospitals it supported to the Syrian government and its Russian allies—even though it had no ability to verify its sources of information or to precisely attribute responsibility for the strikes to one side or another. As a result, these MSF communications have been manipulated by local parties present on the ground, helping them to disseminate unverified and often distorted information. This has, of course, negatively affected MSF's chances of receiving Syrian government authorization to work officially in the country, because the state perceives MSF's communications as unreliable and antigovernment.

THE ROLE OF THE MESSENGER: HOW NUANCE IS LOST

Let's now look at several important cases in which humanitarian NGOs' communications were manipulated.

Hospital Bombings

Médecins Sans Frontières projects in opposition-held areas of Syria consist of two types of programs: MSF-run and MSF-supported. All hospitals run directly by MSF—six at the peak, in 2013, three in mid-2020—were located close to the Turkish border. Because these hospitals were directly run and managed by MSF, the group could follow its usual practice of providing locations (GPS coordinates) to all warring parties with aerial capacity (Syria, Russia, Turkey, Israel, and the US-led coalition). Throughout the conflict, these MSF-run hospitals did not experience bombardments or other aerial attacks (interview with MSF staff). But the big question is, why did they remain untouched? Was it because MSF shared coordinates with all parties to the conflict? Or was it because these hospitals were located close to the Syrian-Turkish border, a de facto no-fly zone? Outside opposition-controlled areas, MSF also had projects and hospitals in the Kurdish regions, run by MSF national and international staff, with MSF staff present on the ground. These hospitals also were not bombed, which is largely explained by the absence of aerial attacks in the Kurdish areas (until Turkey began military operations in the northeastern border regions of Syria, in 2019).

The second type of MSF operations in Syria are support programs, located deeper inside opposition-held areas. In this case MSF doesn't run hospitals and can't operate according to its more common strategies. Such programs consist of providing medical supplies, logistical supplies (including fuel), staff salaries, and training for hospitals and health centers run by others (and often supported by others as well). At the peak of these programs, in 2013–2014, MSF supported around seventy hospitals; by mid-2020 it was about twenty hospitals. Although these hospitals were not MSF-run, the organization offered to include their GPS coordinates in its regular contacts with all warring parties. Yet the managers of these hospitals consistently declined the offer. Many of these hospitals were bombed, some repeatedly.

All MSF communications about the bombings of hospitals in Syria were about these MSF-supported, not MSF-run, hospitals. And because these hospitals often were not marked—and their GPS coordinates not shared— MSF could never communicate that they were intentionally targeted, given that attackers could argue that they did not know they were hospitals. This is why in its communications MSF often describes attacks on hospitals as "indiscriminate attacks on civilian infrastructure including hospitals." But in many cases the original communication is simplified by the media, and the nuance of this message is lost. As a result, MSF has contributed to the narrative that hospitals are intentionally targeted, and that this targeting has been largely carried out by the Syrian government and its Russian allies.

Alleged Chemical Weapon Attack, 2013

In 2013, MSF supported projects and medical facilities in the opposition-controlled enclave in the Damascus suburb of East Ghouta. Important to underline is that this is an example in which no MSF staff members were present on the ground. From a distance, MSF provided technical advice, supplies, money for payroll, fuel, and other logistical support, but those projects were run and managed by local entities.

According to the interviews conducted with MSF staff, on August 21, 2013, facilities in East Ghouta received an influx of patients with symptoms consistent with chemical weapon exposure. During that day, MSF staff and doctors were in contact with the hospitals via a video link that allowed them to observe the situation. The absence of MSF staff on the ground caused a dilemma—whether to speak out about this case or not—and fierce discussions among the internal MSF ranks. There was a significant fear that any MSF communication about this attack would be manipulated (interviews with MSF staff). Eventually, MSF released a cautiously worded statement from its director of operations, avoiding any affirmative sentences about the nature of the attack (chemical or not) or who was responsible (not assigning blame):

> MSF can neither scientifically confirm the cause of these symptoms nor establish who is responsible for the attack. However, the reported symptoms of the patients, in addition to the epidemiological pattern of the events, . . . strongly indicate mass exposure to a neurotoxic agent. This would constitute a violation

of international humanitarian law, which absolutely prohibits the use of chemical and biological weapons. (MSF 2013)

As expected, this MSF press release was immediately picked up by the US State Department, and John Kerry, then the US secretary of state, referred[16] to it when saying that Damascus was behind the chemical attack. This led to a big, unstoppable wave of disinformation, which created a specific, affirmative narrative without an independent investigation or due process. MSF issued a second statement (MSF USA 2013) warning that its medical information could not be used as evidence to certify the precise origin of the exposure to a neurotoxic agent, nor to attribute responsibility. But this statement went largely unnoticed, and it did not help to stop an overwhelming media campaign. This case shows how easily humanitarian INGOs' communications can be manipulated to support another party's argument or policy.

Battle for Aleppo

Another important case in which the humanitarian narrative was manipulated in Syria was the battle for Aleppo (July 2012–December 2016). In this instance, there appeared to be a strong disconnect between the humanitarian rhetoric during the battle, and the actual situation found on the ground after the siege of East Aleppo was over and UN and ICRC workers entered those parts of the city once it was under government control.

From 2012 to 2016, East Aleppo was under the control of armed opposition groups (including the al-Qaeda-affiliated Jabhat al-Nusra), while the rest of the city was under government control. By the fall of 2016, both sides had regularly fired on each other. Back then about 1.5 million people lived in government-held areas, and about three hundred thousand in East Aleppo. The most active phase of the battle lasted from September to December 2016, when both parties attacked, leading to a difficult humanitarian situation. The dominant narrative produced in the global media was that opposition-held East Aleppo was in a desperate humanitarian situation because of a Syrian-Russian-Iranian siege, involving indiscriminate aerial bombardment, which stopped on October 18, 2016, according to Khodinskaya-Golenisheva (2017, 23), but which the UN Security Council reported to continue up to December 9, 2016 (UNSC 2016). Almost all humanitarian agencies relied on information coming from their relief-worker networks inside East Aleppo, meaning that it was almost impossible to independently verify information. Even the United Nations, usually present on both sides, was involved in reproducing information from others, because it had no presence on the ground.

During the battle for East Aleppo, MSF, other humanitarian agencies, and the UN were vocal and critical in their communications about the dire humanitarian situation, the lack of humanitarian access, and indiscriminate Syrian and Russian bombings. They also argued that all hospitals in the area were destroyed, and that medical supplies were running out. Interestingly, many humanitarian organizations stated that there were few hospitals in eastern Aleppo; some said there were no hospitals at all (WHO 2016) and only a handful of doctors who could perform surgeries. Many INGOs simultaneously insisted that supplies of medical equipment be delivered to the besieged part of the city for surgeries and other medical needs (HRW 2016, Islamic Relief 2016). Who was meant to conduct surgeries in an area with few or no hospitals, or enough qualified doctors, remained unclear. Ultimately, MSF and other INGOs—for example, the Syrian American Medical Society (SAMS)—took the opportunity of a moment when the siege was broken to deliver aid to areas of East Aleppo. At that point, the opposition briefly controlled the road to Turkey, bypassing the Syrian government and its Russian allies, which Damascus has used as another argument against working with MSF (interviews with MSF staff).

But when the battle was over, it appeared that the humanitarian situation and the scale of humanitarian need in East Aleppo had been exaggerated to manipulate media coverage, as well as the political stance of many actors and organizations opposed to Syrian and Russian conduct. After the Syrian Arab Army recaptured the eastern part of the city, it reported finding large stockpiles of humanitarian aid, food, medical equipment, and drugs[17] (including supplies with stickers from SAMS, MSF, and the UN) in warehouses under the control of armed groups, including those listed as terrorists. That information was confirmed by a number of UN officials, and by representatives of foreign delegations able to visit the eastern part of Aleppo.[18] The reports spoke of there being enough medical supplies and equipment to address the humanitarian needs of the trapped civil population for months. This aid, however, did not reach many of those in need—about 275,000 people (Khodinskaya-Golenisheva 2017, 43).

Just days after East Aleppo was recaptured by the Syrian army, some international humanitarian organizations started to change their rhetoric about East Aleppo and to criticize its opposition "defenders." The UN High Commissioner for Human Rights for the first time in months voiced concerns about the actions in Aleppo of the Fatah al-Sham Front (affiliated with al-Qaeda):

During the last two weeks, Fatah al-Sham Front and the Abu Amara Battalion are alleged to have abducted and killed an unknown number of civilians who requested the armed groups to leave their neighborhoods, to spare the lives of civilians. . . . We have also received reports that between 30 November and 1 December, armed opposition groups fired on civilians attempting to leave [eastern Aleppo]. (Fisk 2016)

It also appeared that armed groups in East Aleppo had used civilians as human shields; used civilian buildings for military purposes; monopolized food, humanitarian aid, and medical supplies; and suppressed protests of civilians against them (Scherling 2019). In January 2017, the UN secretary-general's report (UN Security Council 2016) also confirmed crimes committed by nonstate armed groups in East Aleppo.

The case of East Aleppo shows how the UN and humanitarian organizations contributed to the dissemination of distorted information. Reproducing information from East Aleppo, with no ability to independently verify it, seriously affected the narrative about the real situation.

It is important to note how the battle for Aleppo compares with the battle for Mosul (2016–2017) conducted by the US-led coalition against ISIS in Iraq, as it shows how differently two almost identical military situations were portrayed and presented to the public. In both situations, a city, or parts of a city, were captured by Islamist armed groups, designated as terrorists by the opposing party; offensives to "liberate" those parts were conducted; heavy artillery and air bombings were used in both cases, leading to immense destruction; and offenders in both cases were government forces supported by international forces and pro-government militias. The difference, however, in how the two episodes were reported and covered in the Western media was huge. In the case of Mosul, Iraqi government forces, pro-government militias, and the US-led anti-ISIS coalition were portrayed as being on "the right side of history," fighting against ISIS "terrorists" who controlled Mosul (Williams and Souza 2017) and about 1.5 million civilians (Lafta, Al-Nuaimi, and Burnham 2018; *Telegraph* 2016). Yet the Syrian Army and its allies' actions, including indiscriminate bombings, were predominantly portrayed as an offensive against the civilian population, not as a fight against "terrorists," even though many armed groups in East Aleppo were designated by the UN and Western states as terrorists and some were affiliated with al-Qaeda. Although in each battle about forty thousand civilians died, those in Mosul were largely portrayed as collateral damage inevitable in a fight against terrorism. Attribution of responsibility in the case of Mosul was less explicitly assigned to those responsible, unless ISIS fighters were clearly behind casualties. But in Aleppo, the attribution of responsibility was so strongly assigned to government forces that it implied the Syrian government and its allies were behind all the deaths there (Scherling 2019).

Another interesting difference is the way humanitarians approached the battles and their work. During the battle for Mosul, humanitarian INGOs worked in close coordination with Iraqi government forces, their allies, and the US-led anti-ISIS coalition, but were absent from ISIS-held areas, as ISIS had denied all access. The situation was quite the opposite in Aleppo, where the majority of humanitarians did not receive permission to work in areas controlled by Syrian government forces, while access to besieged areas was granted by armed opposition groups. According to MSF staff on the ground in Mosul, MSF was in a way trapped, because the only way to work there was by working with the government and the US-led anti-ISIS coalition (interviews with MSF staff). Consequently, in both cases—Aleppo and Mosul—informational narratives were created with the help of respected international humanitarians who relied on one-sided sources who produced a distorted image in order to manipulate both the humanitarians and the media. In the case of Mosul, an MSF staff member stated that humanitarian INGOs and UN agencies have become "force multipliers" for Iraqi government and US forces—that is, a component of the offenders' military strategy—leaving no space for independence and basic medical ethics. If you apply the Mosul logic to Aleppo, a question arises: Would the UN, WHO, or international donors have funded Russian medical posts to be embedded with Syrian Army units during the East Aleppo offensive? The answer seems crystal clear—they would not have (Whittall 2017). Yet in Iraq, humanitarians made this compromise and embedded with one side of the conflict. One MSF staff member who worked in Mosul observed:

> The decisions of WHO and others in how they work in Iraq are not simply about pragmatically getting as close as possible to the frontlines. These decisions are rooted in donor priorities and a political willingness to align healthcare as part of the battle against the Islamic State. The risks of this approach are clear: if doctor and fighter are seen as one, who can patients trust? (Whittall 2017)

THE CHALLENGES AHEAD

The dire security situation in Syria throughout the conflict kept many INGOs and major media outlets from gaining first-hand access to information from all parties of the conflict. Naturally, this situation created a hunger for such information, and in many cases INGOs and the media put their trust in reports coming from local sources in areas under control of armed opposition groups. This absence of ground presence accelerated from 2015 onward, after a wave of abductions of aid workers and journalists.

At the same time, over the years, INGOs have acquired more tools and influence, and they have become more important actors in the realm of information coming from conflict areas. As a result, their capacity to influence external parties to the conflict—regional and international actors— has grown, through their ability to produce and spread (sometimes intentionally, sometimes inadvertently) certain narratives about parties to the conflict through (digital) media. As such, INGOs have become part of the "information warfare" system. This is why INGOs' communications policies and the way these organizations treat and verify information sources should be analyzed more extensively and, where necessary, revised. This will help to decrease the risk of manipulation, as well as the risk of disseminating disinformation that may have serious consequences for the people living in conflict areas.

Humanitarian INGOs are faced with a set of information challenges. Should they report on incidents that cannot be independently and scientifically verified? How should they cover and present their interactions with parties to the conflict while preserving access to populations in need? How should they respond to the instrumentalization of their words by parties to the conflict? And how best should they balance these narratives—these competing points of view of different parties—to ensure their ability to perform their necessary humanitarian work and to ensure their access to populations in need? Answering these questions will help to minimize risks of humanitarian aid being manipulated for political reasons and also will help to change the attitude of warring parties to the work humanitarian NGOs are doing.

Because of the existing challenges and problems around humanitarian NGOs' work in conflict areas, a set of certain engagement rules could be introduced. One of the major points of discussion could be a form of regulation of humanitarian activities of at least those INGOs who work with the UN in conflict areas and/or with the parties of a conflict. For instance, in order to avoid INGOs picking sides in the conflict and to adhere better to the principle of neutrality, INGOs may be obliged to be randomly allocated to specific areas within a conflict zone. In such a system, if humanitarian organizations want to work in a particular country, they would undergo a process that would grant them legitimate rights to operate in an allocated area of that country. This approach might help to avoid INGOs being one-sided while operating in conflict areas. Also, it might even help to increase humanitarian coverage of the population in need with the necessary aid.

This approach also would contribute to balancing different information narratives, which, in turn, will help to decrease manipulation of humanitarian aid through dissemination of disinformation.

NOTES

1. For example, the Anti-Slavery Society, the World Alliance of YMCAs, the International Red Cross and Red Crescent Movement.
2. Consultative Status to the United Nations Economic and Social Council (ECOSOC) is granted by the UN to NGOs and allows them to participate in UN work.
3. See Chapter 5 of this volume by Duncan McLean.
4. As per Inter-Agency Standing Committee, "People in need" refers to people whose physical security, basic rights, dignity, living conditions, or livelihoods are threatened or have been disrupted, and whose current level of access to basic services, goods, and protection is inadequate to re-establish normal living conditions within their accustomed means without assistance. https://humanitarian.atlassian.net/wiki/spaces/imtoolbox/pages/488734850/People+in+Need+PIN+Process.
5. https://www.state.gov/caesar-syria-civilian-protection-act/.
6. See Chapter 5 of this volume by Duncan McLean.
7. USAID, "Statement by Deputy Spokesperson Tom Babington on Funding for the White Helmets," June 14, 2018, https://www.usaid.gov/news-information/press-releases/jun-14-2018-statement-deputy-spokesperson-tom-babington-funding-white-helmets.
8. UK government summary document, 2017, https://assets.publishing.service.gov.uk/government/uploads/system/uploads/attachment_data/file/630409/Syria_Resilience_2017.pdf.
9. From the annex to a May 10, 2017, letter from P. Iliichev, chargé d'affaires a.i. of the Permanent Mission of the Russian Federation to the United Nations, to the UN Secretary-General. The annex, "Syria—Six Years On: From Destruction to Reconstruction. The White Helmets: Fact or Fiction—Intervention by Vanessa Beeley 5/4/2017," is a letter from Beeley, an investigative journalist based in France, describing her investigation into the White Helmets. https://undocs.org/pdf?symbol=en/A/71/910.
10. Ibid.
11. UK government summary document, 2017, https://assets.publishing.service.gov.uk/government/uploads/system/uploads/attachment_data/file/630409/Syria_Resilience_2017.pdf.
12. قوات دفاع مدني السوري, http://www.mod.gov.sy/index.php?node=554&cat=3251.
13. "О предоставлении Международной организации гражданской обороны (МОГО) статуса наблюдателя в Генеральной Ассамблее ООН," Ministry of Foreign Affairs of the Russian Federation, October 28, 2015, https://www.mid.ru/ru/international_organizations/-/asset_publisher/km9HkaXMTium/content/id/1905294
14. "Всемирный день гражданской обороны," Interview with deputy head of Civil Defence directorate of Russian Emergency Ministry in Astrakhan region, March 1, 2018, https://30.mchs.gov.ru/deyatelnost/press-centr/intervyu/2205345

15. Dr. Natalie Roberts, interview by Médecins Sans Frontières, March 13, 2015, https://www.youtube.com/watch?v=4oQVUssxK-U.
16. "Transcript: Secretary of State John Kerry's remarks on alleged Syria chemical attack," *Washington Post,* August 26, 2013, https://www.washingtonpost.com/world/national-security/transcript-secretary-of-state-john-kerrys-remarks-on-alleged-syria-chemical-attack/2013/08/26/40b0b4ea-0e8b-11e3-bdf6-e4fc677d94a1_story.html.
17. "Comment by Foreign Ministry Spokeswoman Maria Zakharova on medical supplies in east Aleppo," Ministry of Foreign Affairs of the Russian Federation, February 6, 2017, https://www.mid.ru/audio/-/asset_publisher/OKaclawz2ZSh/content/id/2628457?p_p_id=101_INSTANCE_OKaclawz2ZSh&_101_INSTANCE_OKaclawz2ZSh_languageId=en_GB.
18. Ibid.

REFERENCES

Amnesty International. 2011a. "Security Council and Arab League Must Act Decisively on Libyan Crimes Today." Press Release February 22, 2011. https://www.amnesty.org/en/press-releases/2011/02/security-council-and-arab-league-must-act-decisively-libyan-crimes-today-20/;

Amnesty International. 2011b "Security Council must refer Libya to International Criminal Court." Press Release, February 25, 2011. https://www.amnesty.org/en/press-releases/2011/02/security-council-must-refer-libya-international-criminal-court/.

Amnesty International. 2011c. "Libya: Organization Calls for Immediate Arms Embargo and Assets Freeze." Press Release February 23, 2011. https://www.amnestyusa.org/press-releases/libya-organization-calls-for-immediate-arms-embargo-and-assets-freeze/

Amnesty International. 2012. "Syria: Fresh Evidence of Armed Forces' Ongoing Crimes Against Humanity." https://www.amnesty.org/en/latest/news/2012/06/syria-fresh-evidence-armed-forces-ongoing-crimes-against-humanity/

Anderson, Mary. 1996. "Humanitarian NGOs in Conflict Intervention." In *Managing Global Chaos: Sources of and Responses to International Conflict,* edited by Chester A. Crocker, Fen Osler Hampson, and Pamela Aall. Washington, DC: United States Institute of Peace.

Anderson, Mary. 1999. *Do No Harm: How Aid Can Support Peace—or War.* Boulder, CO: Lynne Rienner.

Barnett, Michael. 2005. "Humanitarianism Transformed." *Perspectives on Politics* 3 (4): 723–40. doi:10.1017/S1537592705050401.

Beeley, Vanessa. 2015a. "Syria's White Helmets: War by Way of Deception—Part I." *21st Century Wire.* http://21stcenturywire.com/2015/10/23/syrias-white-helmets-war-by-way-of- deception-part-1/.

Beeley, Vanessa. 2015b. "Part II—Syria's White Helmets: War By Way of Deception—'Moderate Executioners." *21st Century Wire.* https://21stcenturywire.com/2015/10/28/part-ii-syrias-white-helmets-war-by-way-of-deception-moderate-executioners/.

Bellin, Eva. 2004. "The Robustness of Authoritarianism in the Middle East: Exceptionalism in Comparative Perspective." *Comparative Politics* 36 (2).

Ben-Ari, Rephael Harel. 2013. *The Legal Status of International Non-Governmental Organizations: Analysis of Past and Present Initiatives (1912–2012).* Leiden: Martinus Nijhoff.

The Borgen Project. 2016. "Top 5 Humanitarian Aid Organizations." https://borgenproject.org/5-top-humanitarian-aid-organizations/.

Cooley, Alexander, and James Ron. 2002. "The NGO Scramble: Organizational Insecurity and the Political Economy of Transnational Action." *International Security* 27 (1): 5–39. www.jstor.org/stable/3092151.

Craddick, William. 2017. "US-Supported Syrian White Helmets Involved with War Crimes Committed by Rebel Groups." ZeroHedge. https://www.zerohedge.com/news/2017-01-20/us-supported-syrian-white-helmets-involved-war-crimes-committed-rebel-groups.

Darden, Jessica. 2019. "Aid to Syria Now Means Abetting Assad." American Enterprise Institute. https://www.aei.org/foreign-and-defense-policy/aid-to-syria-now-means-abetting-assad/.

Dupuy, Kendra, and Siri Aas Rustad. 2018. "Trends in Armed Conflict, 1946–2017." *Conflict Trends 5.* Peace Research Institute Oslo. https://www.prio.org/utility/DownloadFile.ashx?id=1698&type=publicationfile.

Fisk, Robert. 2016. "There Is More Than One Truth to Tell in the Heartbreaking Story of Aleppo." *Independent.* https://www.independent.co.uk/voices/aleppo-falls-to-syrian-regime-bashar-al-assad-rebels-uk-government-more-than-one-story-robert-fisk-a7471576.html.

Håvard, Strand, Siri Aas Rustad, Henrik Urdal, and Håvard Mokleiv Nygård. 2019. "Trends in Armed Conflict, 1946–2018." *Conflict Trends 3.* Peace Research Institute Oslo. https://www.prio.org/utility/DownloadFile.ashx?id=1858&type=publicationfile.

Hayward (blog). https://timhayward.wordpress.com/2017/01/23/amnesty-internationals-war-crimes-in-syria/.

Heller, Sam and Cambanis Thanassis. 2018. "Managing Syrian Conflict May Be Possible. Resolving It Isn't." The Century Foundation. https://tcf.org/content/report/managing-syrian-conflict-may-possible-resolving-isnt/?session=1.

House of Commons Foreign Affairs Committee. 2016. "Libya: Examination of Intervention and Collapse and the UK's Future Policy Options." https://publications.parliament.uk/pa/cm201617/cmselect/cmfaff/119/11902.htm.

Humanitarian Needs Overview. 2019. "Humanitarian Needs Overview: Syrian Arab Republic." https://hno-syria.org/data/downloads/en/full_hno_2019.pdf.

Khodinskaya-Golenisheva, Maria. 2017. *Алеппо: война и дипломатия.* ОЛМА Медиа групп.

HRW (Human Rights Watch). 2016. "Syria: Urgent Need for Aleppo Aid Access." https://www.hrw.org/news/2016/12/12/syria-urgent-need-aleppo-aid-access.

Islamic Relief. 2016. "Urgent Need for Health and Sanitation Support in Aleppo." https://www.islamic-relief.org/urgent-need-health-sanitation-support-aleppo/

Knox Clarke, Paul. 2018. "The State of the Humanitarian System 2018." ALNAP. https://sohs.alnap.org/help-library/the-state-of-the-humanitarian-system-2018-full-report.

Kovalik, Dan. 2012. "Libya and the West's Human Rights Hypocrisy." Huffpost. https://www.huffpost.com/entry/human-rights-libya_b_2001880?_guc_consent_skip=1604357427.

Krieger, Joel, ed. 2001. *The Oxford Companion to Politics of the World.* New York: Oxford University Press.

Lafta R, Al-Nuaimi MA, Burnham G. 2018. "Injury and Death during the ISIS Occupation of Mosul and Its Liberation: Results from a 40- Cluster Household Survey. *PLoS Med* 15(5): e1002567. https://doi.org/10.1371/journal.pmed.1002567.

Lebedeva, Marina M., and Maxim V. Kharkevich. 2013. *Негосударственные участники мировой политики*. Аспект Пресс.

Lund, Aron. 2018. "As Syria Looks to Rebuild, US and Allies Hope Money Can Win Where Guns Lost." The New Humanitarian. https://www.thenewhumanitarian.org/analysis/2018/05/22/syria-looks-rebuild-us-and-allies-hope-money-can-win-where-guns-lost.

Marsden, Peter. 1997. "Afghanistan: State Disintegration and the Role of NGOs." In *NGOs and Governments: A Review of Current Practice for Southern and Eastern NGOs*, edited by Jon Bennett. Oxford: INTRAC.

Mason, Jake. 2017. "Power, Petroleum, and Propaganda: Identifying the Role of the White Helmets in the Syrian Civil War" (master's dissertation). University of Sheffield.

McMahon, Patrice. 2017. *The NGO Game: Post-Conflict Peacebuilding in the Balkans and Beyond*. Ithaca, NY: Cornell University Press.

Morningstar, Cory. 2014. "Syria: Avaaz, Purpose, and the Art of Selling Empire." Wrong Kind of Green (blog). http://www.wrongkindofgreen.org/2014/09/17/syria-avaaz-purpose-the-art-of-selling-hate-for-empire/.

MSF (Médecins Sans Frontières). 2004. "Rwandan Refugee Camps in Zaire and Tanzania 1994–1995." MSF Speaking Out. https://www.msf.org/speakingout/rwandan-refugee-camps-zaire-and-tanzania-1994-1995.

MSF (Médecins Sans Frontières). 2013. "Thousands Suffering Neurotoxic Symptoms Treated in Hospitals Supported by MSF." https://www.msf.org/syria-thousands-suffering-neurotoxic-symptoms-treated-hospitals-supported-msf.

MSF (Médecins Sans Frontières). 2016. "Hospitals Hit Repeatedly by Russian and Syrian Airstrikes, Condemning Hundreds of Wounded to Certain Death." https://www.msf.org/syria-hospitals-hit-repeatedly-russian-and-syrian-airstrikes-condemning-hundreds-wounded-certain.

MSF (Médecins Sans Frontières). 2020. "Horrific Day of Indiscriminate Attacks on Civilians in Idlib, Syria." https://www.msf.org/horrific-day-indiscriminate-attacks-idlib-syria.

MSF USA (Médecins Sans Frontières/Doctors Without Borders). 2013. "Response to Government References to MSF Syria Statement." https://www.doctorswithoutborders.org/what-we-do/news-stories/news/response-government-references-msf-syria-statement.

Paul, James A. 2000. "NGOs and Global Policy-Making." Global Policy Forum. https://www.globalpolicy.org/empire/31611-ngos-and-global-policy-making.html.

Robinson, Piers. 2002. *The CNN Effect: The Myth of News, Foreign Policy, and Intervention*. London and New York: Routledge.

Scherling, Johannes. 2019. "A Tale of Two Cities: A Comparative Study of Media Narratives of the Battles for Aleppo and Mosul." *Media, War & Conflict*. doi: 10.1177/1750635219870224.

Shaheen, Kareem. 2016. "Airstrikes Hit Two Syrian Hospitals, with Turkey Condemning 'Obvious War Crime.'" *Guardian*, Feb. 15, 2016. https://www.theguardian.com/world/2016/feb/15/airstrike-destroys-msf-clinic-northern-syria.

Simons, Greg. 2019. "Syria: Propaganda as a Tool in the Arsenal of Information Warfare." In *The SAGE Handbook of Propaganda*, edited by Paul Baines, Nicholas O'Shaughnessy, and Nancy Show. London: SAGE.

Start Network. 2013. "The Future of Non-Governmental Organisations in the Humanitarian Sector." Humanitarian Futures Programme Discussion Paper for the Start Network. https://startnetwork.org/resource/future-non-governmental-organisations-humanitarian-sector.

Stephenson, Max, and Laura Zanotti. 2012. *Peacebuilding Through Community-Based NGOs: Paradoxes and Possibilities*. Sterling, VA: Kumarian Press.

Taylor, Adam. 2014. "Gaddafi Died 3 Years Ago. Would Libya Be Better Off If He Hadn't?" *Washington Post*. https://www.huffpost.com/entry/human-rights-libya_b_2001880?_guc_consent_skip=1604357427.

The Telegraph. 2016. "What Is the Battle for Mosul? Everything You Need to Know About the Fight to Liberate ISIL's Last Bastion of Power in Iraq." https://www.telegraph.co.uk/news/2016/10/17/what-is-the-battle-for-mosul-isils-last-bastion-of-power-in-iraq/

UN General Assembly. 2005. "Resolution Adopted By the General Assembly on 16 September 2005." https://www.un.org/en/development/desa/population/migration/generalassembly/docs/globalcompact/A_RES_60_1.pdf.

UN Security Council. 2016. "Implementation of Security Council Resolutions 2139 (2014), 2165 (2014), 2191 (2014), 2258 (2015) and 2332 (2016), Report of the Secretary-General." https://undocs.org/en/S/2017/58.

Whittall, Jonathan. 2017. "Medics as Force Multipliers Around Mosul—At the Expense of Medical Ethics?" BMJ Opinion. https://blogs.bmj.com/bmj/2017/06/14/medics-as-force-multipliers-around-mosul-at-the-expense-of-medical-ethics/.

WHO. 2016. "Eastern Aleppo Without Any Hospitals for More Than 250,000 Residents." https://www.who.int/news-room/detail/20-11-2016-eastern-aleppo-without-any-hospitals-for-more-than-250-000-residents.

Williams, Brian, and Robert Souza. 2017. "The Fall of a Jihadist Bastion: A History of the Battle of Mosul (October 2016–July 2017)." The Jamestown Foundation. *Terrorism Monitor* 15(19). https://jamestown.org/program/fall-jihadist-bastion-history-battle-mosul-october-2016-july-2017/.

Zonova, Tatiana. 2013. "Will NGOs Survive in the Future?" Russian International Affairs Council. https://russiancouncil.ru/en/analytics-and-comments/analytics/will-ngos-survive-in-the-future/.

CHAPTER 8

Naming and Shaming the Bombers

MICHIEL HOFMAN

The bombing of hospitals has occurred throughout the history of wars, by accident or design. The series of Geneva Conventions, from their first version in 1864 onward, tried to award some protection to "the medical mission" and may have reduced the practice, but it has certainly not been eliminated. Humanitarian organizations such as Médecins Sans Frontières (MSF), claiming protection under these conventions, still find themselves in the crosshairs of such attacks.

In the Syrian conflict, in the second decade of the twenty-first century, the frequency of such events appears to have increased dramatically (Briody et al. 2018). The years 2015 and 2016 stand out as particularly volatile. In a thirteen-month period, *The Lancet* recorded a peak in attacks in Syria, with 402 attacks on 135 health facilities (Elamein et al. 2017). In Yemen, the World Health Organization (WHO) reported 102 health facilities damaged or destroyed in a seventeen-month period.[1] And in Afghanistan, the October 2015 bombing of an MSF trauma hospital in Kunduz stood out for its sheer violence and brutality: forty-two people were killed, including twenty-four patients, and thirty-seven people were injured.[2]

These three wars, in which the hospital bombings were committed by major world powers such as the United States and Russia, and by regional powers such as Saudi Arabia, brought the phenomenon to the forefront of the public consciousness for a brief time. This global attention was driven partly by sustained "naming and shaming" campaigns by humanitarian organizations, including MSF, which in the hope of putting an end to the

Michiel Hofman, *Naming and Shaming the Bombers* In: *Everybody's War*. Edited by: Jehan Bseiso,
Michiel Hofman, and Jonathan Whittall, Oxford University Press. © Médecins Sans Frontières 2021.
DOI: 10.1093/oso/9780197514641.003.0009

practice identified perpetrators and accused them of breaching international humanitarian law—effectively a war crime (International Committee
of the Red Cross, Health Care in Danger,[3] MSF, Medical Care Under Fire,[4]
Safeguarding Health in Conflict 2017, SAMS 2017, WHO 2016).

Globally, the number of bombings has since diminished,[5] perhaps as a
result of these campaigns. But especially in Syria the naming and shaming
does not appear to have had any effect (PHR 2019). A closer look at the history of hospital bombings, the mechanics of naming and shaming, and the
specificity of the Syrian conflict gives some clues as to why this is the case.
Specifically, MSF's use of naming and shaming between 2014 and 2016
reveals some of the dilemmas that have rendered the practice in Syria less
effective.

HISTORICAL LIMITATIONS OF THE GENEVA CONVENTIONS

The Geneva Conventions have never prevented attacks on medical facilities.
Since the first "Geneva Convention for the Amelioration of the Condition of
the Wounded in Armies in the Field" in 1864,[6] warring parties have violated
the protections the conventions award to their enemies and abused the
conventions' terms for their own military advantage. The first "test" of the
conventions, during the Franco-Prussian War of 1870–1871, already saw
warring parties denying their own violations and accusing their enemies of
abusing the regulations, as well as the associated symbol of the red cross
flags marking immunity from attack for military gain (McLean 2019). The
nature of humanitarianism, the Geneva Conventions, and how they were
violated are distinct before, during, and after the Cold War.

A striking example of the early period is the rhetoric used by Italy
during the Italo-Ethiopian War of 1935–1937, after seventeen attacks on
Red Cross hospitals, seven by "direct bombings." Italy initially denied the
damage, changed official flight reports to accommodate that claim, and
shifted the blame to the Ethiopians by asserting that "everything was
covered in Red-Cross signs including army camps and even the airfield"
(McLean 2019). The Geneva Conventions before the Second World War
were still limited to medical care in conflict, coinciding with the period
that humanitarian assistance was closely linked with the colonial period,
in what the political scientist Michael Barnett calls the first age of humanitarianism (Barnett 2011).

The 1949 Geneva Conventions, although extending their reach to general protection of civilian populations, did not stop the practice of hospital bombings. The Nigerian government repeated the strategy of denying

and deferring blame during the Nigerian Civil War of 1967–1970; in that war, the International Committee of the Red Cross (ICRC) recorded sixteen instances in which medical structures were bombed. The Nigerians, although apologetic, went from blaming "poor weather" for the "mistake" to outright accusing the Biafran rebels of taking advantage of the Red Cross to secure their military assets. The Nigerian government claimed at the time that "secessionists [were] using hospitals and other protected sites to store arms, munitions and troops," and that it was a "deliberate policy of the rebels" to hide themselves in populated areas. These rhetorical tactics from states are similar to those used by governments in Syria, Yemen, and Afghanistan today (McLean 2019).

The role of humanitarians was very different in this period, however. During the Cold War (1947–1991) there was an interval of rapid growth in both the number and size of independent humanitarian organizations, mostly founded, based, and funded in Western Europe and North America. Unsurprisingly, the rise of Western humanitarianism and Western Cold War foreign policy objectives often colluded with each other.[7] Barnett calls this the second age of humanitarianism, defined mostly by the East–West divide (Barnett 2011). Alignment with Cold War objectives can lead to humanitarian organizations themselves compromising the very principles of international humanitarian law (IHL) designed to allow humanitarians to operate. The former director of the MSF Switzerland research unit, Caroline Abu Sa'da, notes that historically MSF has been one of the organizations making these compromises on its principles:

> From the Vietnam War to the conflicts in Afghanistan against the Soviet invaders, humanitarian involvement in the Cold War did not always abide by the principles of neutrality and impartiality. Instead, humanitarian personnel acted in accordance with other, more partisan considerations, often focusing on identifying victims of oppressive regimes, which led them to concentrate their efforts on a particular cause and group. In the operational history of MSF, such choices clearly demonstrate that there is a degree of ambivalence regarding principles when it comes to practice. (Abu Sa'da et al. 2013)

After the Cold War, according to Barnett, humanitarianism transformed itself into a vehicle for spreading liberal democracy and human rights (Barnett 2011). Conflicts also changed, from interstate to intrastate— internal conflicts with parties supported directly or indirectly by other states—and since the early 2000s largely have been conducted with a doctrine of counterinsurgency or counterterrorism. In this environment, attacks on medical structures take place in a context wherein other violations of humanitarian law, such as indiscriminate attacks on civilians, are also commonplace. Abu Sa'da describes the counterinsurgency doctrine as one "which makes the distinction between civilians and combatants (an essential precept of international law) illusory" (Abu Sa'da et al. 2013). In this counterinsurgency logic, attacks on hospitals are just "collateral damage," as a distinction between military and civilian structures can no longer be made, and special protection to wounded enemy combatants can no longer be awarded.

This historical overview of the effectiveness of the Geneva Conventions in protecting medical structures during conflict paints a grim picture, in which IHL looks to become increasingly irrelevant. If since its inception in 1864 the Geneva Convention has been violated by warring parties and by the humanitarians it was supposed to enable during the Cold War, and has now been completely rejected under counterinsurgency doctrine, then the sharp surge in hospital bombings noted between 2015 and 2016 in Syria and Yemen should hardly be a surprise. But at the same time, global attention to the attacks on medics, and the relevance of IHL, has also surged, as citizens, civil society, humanitarians, and international organizations have never been as able to record, report on, and disseminate information on these attacks in such detail, through the Internet and especially social media channels. When similar disregard for medical protection happened during the 1930s, by the Italians during their war with Ethiopia, or during the 1960s, by the Nigerians during the Biafra war, only a handful of specialist diplomats and an occasional journalist took note. The volume of humanitarian deployment in conflict has increased significantly, and with it hospital bombings in Syria, Yemen, and Afghanistan have penetrated the consciousness of a wide general audience. The people now paying attention may not know the intricacies of the Geneva Convention, but they intuitively understand that bombing a building full of sick people is wrong, and conceive of the Geneva Convention, designed to protect them, as "good" and "just."

ATTACKS ON HEALTH CARE AFTER 2010

In the wake of this public attention, studies by academics, humanitarians, and human rights organizations have sought to quantify the reality of hospital attacks—often with the explicit purpose of pressuring the illusive "international community" (such as the United Nations Security Council) to act. Carolyn Briody and colleagues looked into the great conflicts of the 1990s and early 2000s and listed the total number of reports of health facilities attacked (Bosnia: 21, Chechnya: 24, Kosovo: 100) and the conflicts dominating the 2010 decade (Iraq: 12, Syria: 135 or 315, Yemen: 93). They noted that "for many conflicts it is not clear if destruction of facilities is a byproduct of the failure to take precautions required by Geneva Conventions or if attacks were a deliberate strategy" (Briody et al. 2018). When these numbers are broken down to an average number of attacks per month, the outcome does not conclude that the perceived surge in the 2010s is exceptional. Kosovo and Yemen both score high, with 6.67 and 4.65 per month, respectively; Bosnia and Iraq score low, with 0.41 and 0.12 attacks per month; and the second Chechen war falls somewhat in the middle, with 2.4. In this study Syria could be the odd one out, depending on how an attack on a health facility is counted. According to data obtained from Physicians for Human Rights (PHR), Syria had an average of 4.38 attacks per month over a seven-year period; data obtained from the "Health Cluster" based in Turkey—a United Nations–led humanitarian health coordination body—showed an average of 9.64 attacks per month, which would constitute a much higher than "normal" incidence of health center attacks (Briody et al. 2018).

A global report by the World Health Organization (WHO), on attacks on health care in emergencies for 2014–2015, was more conclusive about the exceptionally high number of attacks in Syria. The report recorded 338 attacks in 19 countries in 2014, and 256 attacks in 16 countries in 2015, of which "the Syrian Arab Republic had the most reported attacks on healthcare each year: twice as many attacks as any other country or territory in 2014 and nearly four times as many attacks in 2015" (WHO 2016). This worked out as 28 percent of global incidents taking place in Syria in 2014, and a staggering 53 percent in 2015. The report also noted that roughly two thirds of all cases were reported as intentional but acknowledged that this did not give any indication of the reasons behind the presumed intent, which made these figures somewhat subjective. The WHO also noted that 53 percent of the recorded attacks were reported as perpetrated by states and 30 percent as perpetrated by nonstate actors; the remaining 17 percent were unreported, or perpetrators were undetermined (WHO 2016).

This high level of state complicity in attacks on health care was the focus of a report published by Safeguarding Health in Conflict, an ad-hoc coalition of thirty-six academic, medical, human rights, and humanitarian organizations recording attacks on health care in twenty-three countries in 2016. This was the year in which on May 3 the United Nations Security Council adopted Resolution 2286, on the protection of civilians in armed conflict.[8] The Safeguarding Health report concluded that in 2016, "governments that ignored, denied, or justified attacks on health facilities, potentially involving their military forces, include Afghanistan, Iraq, Israel, Libya, Russia, Saudi Arabia, Sudan, Syria, Ukraine, and the United States," and that "it must be emphasized that in the months since the passing of resolution 2286, attacks on hospitals dramatically escalated in Syria and continued without respite in other parts of the world" (Safeguarding Health in Conflict 2017). The report also concluded that in 2016, "Syria was by far the worst case," with 108 reported attacks; in 90 percent of these attacks, Syria and its (Russian) allies were listed as the perpetrators.

HOSPITAL BOMBINGS IN SYRIA

Physicians for Human Rights documented 553 attacks on at least 348 separate health facilities in 2012–2018, of which 73 were air bombardments (PHR 2019). All but 2 percent of the attacks were attributed to the Syrian government and its allies. The share of aerial attacks increased yearly, from just 38 percent in 2012 to 90 percent in 2018. These were exceptionally high numbers in both historical and geographical perspective. PHR did not hesitate to attribute intentionality behind these attacks:

> The systematic targeting of health facilities has been a crucial component of a wider strategy of war employed by the Syrian government and its allies—who are responsible for over 90 percent of attacks—to punish civilians residing in opposition held territories, destroy their ability to survive, and draw them into government-held areas or drive them out of the country. (PHR 2019)

The Syrian American Medical Society (SAMS), a humanitarian organization based in Turkey with many projects in opposition-held territories in Syria, linked specific events to the acceleration of aerial attacks in 2016. It noted that from January to September 2015, the rate of attacks was one every four days (SAMS 2017). After the Russian air force entered the theater of war in support of the Syrian army, in September 2015, the rate of attacks doubled to one every two days. The offensive on Eastern Aleppo, supported by Syrian and Russian aerial attacks between September and November 2016, resulted in an overall rate of aerial attacks in Syria of one every day.

The Syrian American Medical Society attributed an even higher share of all attacks to Syrian forces and their allies. In 172 attacks recorded in 2015–2016, it pointed to the Syrian-led coalition as the perpetrator in 168 cases, to the armed opposition in two cases, and to two unknowns. SAMS also concluded that attacks on health care were targeted and intentional, a "systematic effort to help cripple neighborhoods and drive displacement, dovetailing with siege warfare tactics" (SAMS 2017). In response to these high levels of attacks, especially since 2015, the Syria Health Cluster based in Turkey asked all its humanitarian partners with medical activities in Syria to participate in a Monitoring Violence Against Health Care (MVH) alert network, in an attempt to comprehensively quantify the problem. This included a record of the human cost of these attacks:

> Between early November 2015, and Dec 31 2016, 938 people were directly harmed in 402 incidents of violence against health care: 677 (72%) were wounded and 261 (28%) were killed. Most of the dead were adult males (68%), but the highest case fatality (39%) was seen in children aged younger than 5 years. 24% of attack victims were health workers. Around 44% of hospitals and 5% of all primary care clinics in mainly areas with a substantial presence of armed opposition groups experienced attacks. Aerial bombardment was the main form of attack. A third of health-care services were hit more than once. Services providing trauma care were attacked more than other services. (Elamein et al. 2017)

However, Elamein and colleagues recognized the limitations of a remote reporting tool lacking oversight from independent researchers. Some of the reporting sources might have had political agendas—with an interest to over-report number of incidents, but also to under-report other aspects, given that not all areas were covered by the participating organizations. This study did not allocate blame, but urged warring parties to respect IHL and international bodies to use their data to hold these parties to account. An analysis by a partnership between *The Lancet* and the American University of Beirut did not hold back in accusing the warring parties, principally the Syrian government, of war crimes. They proposed that the purpose of attacks on hospitals was a military strategy, the "use of violence to restrict or deny access to care as a weapon of war" (Fouad et al. 2017).

This concept of "weaponization" of health care was proposed early in the conflict. In 2012, MSF published a report called "Syria: Medicine as a Weapon of Persecution," documenting the testimonies of fifteen medics at the start of the conflict, when most of the wounded came from street protests violently suppressed by Syrian security forces (MSF 2012). This assertion of the Syrian state intentionally attacking health structures and staff is often attributed to a counterterrorism law adopted by the Syrian parliament in 2012, a law the United Nations Human Rights Council (OHCHR) deemed in violation of IHL, because it "effectively criminalized medical aid to the opposition" (OHCHR 2013).

The sequence of events in Syria, showing a steady increase in the number of attacks on health facilities and in the proportion of attacks by air—the majority of which have been attributed to the Syrian government and its allies—suggests that naming (and shaming) the perpetrators is a straightforward exercise. The analyses conducted by MVH and SAMS, covering a similar period, identify the offensive on East Aleppo in the second half of 2016 as responsible for a major share of the total number of attacks (Elamein 2017, SAMS 2017). Syrian and Russian aircraft relentlessly bombed the neighborhood to rubble, including all functioning health facilities. Many organizations, including MSF, condemned the Syrian government and its allies (naming) for attacking hospitals, blocking medical supplies, and preventing medical evacuations—and for the gross violations of IHL these actions represented (shaming).[9] After the "fall of East Aleppo" in December 2016, when Syrian government forces regained control over the area from armed opposition forces, the OHCHR launched an independent commission of inquiry in response to the sheer brutality of the events. Its report to the United Nations General Assembly (UNGA) revealed the complexity of the environment.

The report did confirm that "between July and December 2016, Syrian and Russian forces carried out daily air strikes, claiming hundreds of lives and reducing hospitals, schools and markets to rubble," but it also noted that "armed groups persistently shelled civilians in western Aleppo city," and that "as the situation deteriorated in eastern Aleppo and people tried desperately to flee, some armed groups violently prevented them and used them as human shields" (UNGA 2017). The report recognized that the military capabilities of the Syrian coalition were much larger than those of the armed opposition and that the level of violence was consequently much higher.

The report also revealed the complex nature of the various armed actors. The Syrian army not only relied on Russian allies in the air, but also on "national militias, such as the Ba'ath Brigades, the Tiger Forces, and the Liwa al-Quds Brigade, as well as members of foreign militias, to increase its ground offensive capacity. These included the Army of the Guardians of the Islamic Revolution (Iran Revolutionary Guards Corps) al-Quds Force, Hezbollah, Afghan militias and the Iraqi al-Nujabaa and al-Fatimiyoon militias (pro-Government forces)." The armed opposition included "Harakat Nour al-Din al-Zenki, Jaish al-Mujahedeen, Aljabha al-Shamiya, Failaq al-Sham, Ahrar as-Sham, Fastaqim Kama Umirt Union and Sultan Murad Brigade, among other factions"—all groups that the report accused of using civilian buildings for military purposes, diverting aid, using civilians as human shields, and intimidating the population generally. This muddle of factions and loyalties on both sides made it difficult to pinpoint responsibility for specific events, other than the aerial bombardments, which were clearly the remit of Syrian/Russian air forces, given that none of the other parties had this capacity. Accordingly, the OHCHR reserved its hardest punches for the Syrian coalition in the air, calling its actions a "war crime of intentionally targeting protected objects" as well as "intentionally attacking medical personnel and transport" (UNGA 2017).

Aerial attacks could be attributed to the Syrian-led coalition because the other air forces deployed in the Syrian airspace, in a US-led counterterrorist coalition, were not active in the skies over Aleppo. Still, the US-led coalition's presence added to the complexity, as its activities elsewhere in the country affected a ceasefire brokered between the United States and Russia on September 13, 2016.[10] A few days later, on September 17, US airplanes struck Syrian army positions near the city of Deir-e-Zour, supposedly aimed at Islamic State (IS) positions—which would have been allowed under the terms of the ceasefire. Yet the Russians accused the United States of deliberately targeting the Syrian army positions, not accepting the US apology.

On September 20, the day the one-week ceasefire came to an end, Syrian coalition planes bombed a UN-led aid convoy to East Aleppo, even though the terms of this convoy were agreed upon in advance by the Syrian government. This event was a defining moment during the battle for East Aleppo. Negotiations for such aid deliveries—and medical evacuations—also involved parties and locations far beyond East Aleppo. Some of the armed opposition groups active in East Aleppo also were involved in the rare occurrence wherein opposition groups besieged towns loyal to the government— two small towns in the Idlib countryside, Foue and Kefraya. Allowing goods into East Aleppo was made conditional on opposition groups also allowing aid into these towns. But the towns "had been tied into a tit-for-tat agreement brokered by the UN, called the 'four towns agreement,' which meant any medical evacuation from one had to be reciprocated with evacuations from the other" (Atlantic Council 2017). This brought two other towns into the fray on the other side of the country close to the Lebanese border, Madaya and Zabadini, which were besieged by Hezbollah, an ally of the Syrian government. The Atlantic Council noted that "the same was true for aid deliveries. Once Foua and Kafraya were in play, Madaya and Zabadani had to be, too. The fate of those in east Aleppo was now tied to four other locations, and theirs, in turn, to the fate of Aleppo." The entanglement continued right till the end: "On the morning of December 18, civilians in Foua and Kafraya waited to leave, as did those in east Aleppo" (Atlantic Council 2017).

MÉDECINS SANS FRONTIÈRES DILEMMAS

The bombing of hospitals as a risk associated with working in warzones is one MSF has experienced for decades. Depending on the political circumstances, MSF has condemned such attacks publicly and, when possible and expedient, has specified which party it holds responsible. Before 2015, such announcements largely went unnoticed outside humanitarian circles and the immediate country or region in which such incidents occurred. For instance, the bombings of MSF hospitals in Sudan in 1999[11] and 2014[12] were largely ignored.

This changed after the bombing of MSF's Kunduz trauma hospital in Afghanistan by US forces in October 2015.[13] The brutality of the attack—sustained bombing targeted specifically at the hospital building, leaving forty-eight people dead, including immobile patients who burned to death in their hospital beds—and the fact that US forces accepted responsibility pushed the topic to the front of the public consciousness. Global news outlets, east and west, north and south, started reporting on hospital bombings in 2015 and 2016 that occurred in Syria and Yemen. This international attention brought international scrutiny to MSF's messaging as well. Why did MSF label the bombing in Afghanistan a war crime, calling for an international investigation, but not the bombings in Yemen and Syria? Why did MSF name the perpetrators in Afghanistan and Yemen, but not in Syria? The people living in Afghanistan, Yemen, and Syria also started to take notice of MSF's discourse after each event. Why did MSF mobilize howls of protest from all over the world and secure a public apology from US President Barack Obama after Kunduz, but seemingly say little and do nothing when Russia bombed hospitals in Syria, or when Saudi Arabia bombed hospitals in Yemen?

Internally, MSF justifies its communications decisions with roughly four objectives: *outrage*, aiming to bear witness and show solidarity with victims; *accountability*, to ensure MSF's actions are transparent; *impunity*, to ensure warring parties pay a political cost; and *leverage*, to reduce the risk of future attacks. Unwritten, but underlying these choices, is the *do no harm* principle. But what if outrage and public shaming make warring parties more aggressive, even more likely to bomb the next hospital? These internal considerations, however, are not useful to justify inconsistencies to the victims or the perpetrators.

Communications are only as useful as their relevance to those who listen to them. This requires the messenger, in this case MSF, to be credible. As a medical organization, MSF starts with an advantage—"everyone trusts doctors"—but this trust can rapidly disappear if the messages are inconsistent or unbelievable.

MÉDECINS SANS FRONTIÈRES LACK OF CONSISTENCY

A review of all of MSF's official press statements[14] after the bombing of its hospitals during the peak years of such attacks (2014–2016) revealed inconsistencies. The analysis looked at whether the press releases named the perpetrators (naming) and whether an accusation was included (shaming). It also looked at the accusations most commonly used by MSF; namely, that an attack did not respect the protection of health facilities in general, that an attack was, in fact, a breach of IHL, and in some cases that the attack was deliberate—targeted—which would indicate a war crime had been committed. The claim that an attack was deliberate is stronger when a hospital is clearly marked, the location of the hospital is known to the warring parties, or both. This element is captured in Table 8.1 as "GPS."

Finally, because MSF works with two different ways of running hospital projects—directly managed by MSF or support to a third-party hospital (usually managed by health ministries)—this is also indicated, because MSF cannot communicate without the consent of such a partner for the supported hospitals. This influences the content of the message.

The single event in Afghanistan in the 2014–2016 period, the Kunduz hospital bombing, stands out not only because of the brutality of the event and the high death toll of forty-eight patients and staff, but also as a case study of the importance of consistency in messaging. The US and Afghan authorities learned this lesson the hard way. MSF gained the edge in public confidence as the facts presented in their public discourse remained consistent, while the United States appeared to change its story several times in the first three days (Bouchet-Saulnier and Whittall 2018). The perceived unreliability of the US and Afghan public response determined the tone of any public discourse around Kunduz. As a result, anything the US government or the Afghan government said about the event was questioned, while MSF was hardly challenged on any of its discourse.

This was one of the main reasons MSF was pressured after October 2015 by its Syrian medical partners, the victims of the bombings, other international organizations, and some of the press to "name and shame" the Russian bombings in Syria. Among others, this inconsistency was seized

Table 8.1. MSF PRESS RELEASES ON HOSPITAL BOMBINGS 2014–2016 NAME AND SHAME PRACTICE

Date	Country	MSF/Supp	GPS	Name	Target	Respect	IHL
2016							
19 Nov	Syria	Supported	No	No	No	Yes	Yes
17 Nov	Syria	Supported	No	No	No	No	No
15 Oct	Syria	Supported	No	Yes	No	No	No
7 Oct	Syria	Supported	No	Yes	Yes	Yes	Yes
7 Oct	Syria	Supported	No	Yes	No	No	No
5 Oct	Syria	Supported	No	Yes	No	No	No
30 Sep	Syria	Supported	No	Yes	No	Yes	No
28 Sep	Syria	Supported	No	No	No	No	No
15 Aug	Yemen	Supported	Yes	Yes	No	Yes	No
8 Aug	Syria	Supported	No	No	Yes	Yes	No
28 Apr	Syria	Supported	No	No	Yes	Yes	No
15 Feb	Syria	Supported	No	No	Yes	No	No
9 Feb	Syria	Supported	No	No	No	Yes	Yes
10 Jan	Yemen	Supported	Yes	No	Yes	Yes	Yes
2015							
3 Dec	Yemen	MSF	Yes	Yes	No	Yes	Yes
1 Dec	Syria	Supported	No	No	Yes	Yes	No
21 Nov	Syria	Supported	No	No	Yes	No	No
27 Oct	Yemen	Supported	Yes	Yes	No	No	Yes
3 Oct	Afghanistan	MSF	Yes	Yes	Yes	Yes	Yes
14 Aug	Syria	Supported	No	Yes	Yes	Yes	N/A
18 June	Syria	Supported	No	No	Yes	Yes	Yes
4 May	Syria	Supported	No	No	Yes	Yes	No
3 Feb	Ukraine	Supported	No	No	No	Yes	No
23 Jan	Ukraine	Supported	No	No	No	Yes	No
20 Jan	Sudan	MSF	Yes	Yes	N/A	No	No
2014							
29 July	Gaza	Supported	N/A	Yes	Yes	Yes	Yes
24 July	Iraq	Supported	No	No	Yes	No	No
28 June	Iraq	MSF	No	No	No	Yes	No
17 Jun	Sudan	MSF	Yes	Yes	No	Yes	No

MSF/Supp: Hospital managed by MSF or MSF supporting non-MSF hospital.
GPS: MSF mentions in press release that GPS coordinates are shared with warring parties.
Name: MSF names the alleged perpetrators of the bombing in the press release.
Target: MSF claims in the press release that the bombing deliberately targeted health facilities.
Respect: MSF calls on warring parties to respect the safety of health facilities.
IHL: MSF accuses the bombers of breaching IHL.

upon by those willing to discredit the accounts of hospital bombings in Syria as proof that MSF was not a reliable witness, notably the Syrian and Russian authorities.[15] Naturally, the attacks on MSF hospitals by two global superpowers and historical Cold War adversaries within months of each other generated public interest, and comparison of MSF's reaction, but these two contexts were not the only ones in which the messaging from MSF was inconsistent.

The analysis of MSF's communications about, in total, twenty-nine hospital bombings in 2014–2016 revealed that MSF did not name the perpetrators of airstrikes in Iraq and Ukraine, but did so in Gaza, Sudan, and most cases in Yemen. In Syria, where MSF-supported hospitals were attacked seventeen times, the perpetrators were named on five occasions. MSF "shamed" on all occasions, but only ten times made the accusation of breach of IHL, nineteen times using the more generic "calling to respect health structures." IHL was not invoked for Sudan, Iraq, or Ukraine. It was invoked for Yemen except on one occasion, and strongly invoked— including a call for an independent investigation by the International Humanitarian Fact Finding Commission (IHFFC)[16]—in Afghanistan and once in Yemen. For Syria, MSF called for respect for IHL on five of seventeen occasions, the same number of times MSF named the perpetrators in Syria, but not about the same events. The decision not to invoke IHL after the attack in Kordofan, Sudan, in 2014, appears the most inconsistent in this respect, because the circumstances in which MSF did invoke the breaching of IHL—in Afghanistan, Gaza, and Yemen—were quite similar, with known, visible structures with GPS locations shared and known perpetrators. Syria stands out, first and foremost because more than half of all hospital attacks in the period analyzed occurred in Syria, but also because MSF's messaging was inconsistent in terms of both naming and shaming *within* the same country.

MÉDECINS SANS FRONTIÈRES AS A CREDIBLE WITNESS

Other factors affect MSF's credibility as a witness. As a medical organization, MSF starts from a good place, first because doctors are almost universally regarded as trustworthy and reliable, although mostly if they speak about medical needs and consequences. However, *which* doctors are speaking makes a difference. Firsthand reports from international medical staff—supposedly because they are not influenced by the local politics, but realistically also because of entrenched colonial attitudes among Western academic, humanitarian, and media institutions—are almost always seen as the most reliable. Medical staff directly employed by MSF are seen as more reliable than local medics supported by MSF.

In this light, there is a clear hierarchy in credibility linked to the MSF statements on hospital bombings in these three years. On top are Gaza, Kunduz, and Yemen, with international, MSF-employed staff directly witnessing the airstrikes; closely behind is Sudan, with MSF national staff. Syria, Iraq, and Ukraine, which were non-MSF facilities supported with medicines and expertise by MSF, are seen as least reliable, because MSF staff members do not witness directly, but relay reports by medical staff they support. This ranking does not indicate how credible MSF regards its own messages to be, or how credible MSF judges its own staff or partners to be. Nor does it say much about how credible journalists, or their readers, find the story, as generally they are not aware of these subtle differences on the ground and simply register that "yet another MSF hospital was bombed."

The credibility of the witness starts to matter, however, because facts and figures are likely to be scrutinized and challenged by those accused of causing the event. The more precise the message on medical data such as numbers of wounded and killed—or on other precisions like the numbers of women and children involved, or why the bombing constitutes a breach of IHL—the less the reliability of the messenger (be it national, international, or partner staff) is questioned.

NAMING

These inconsistencies may seem sloppy or careless, but context is everything. MSF had good reason to name or shame in some cases but not in others. Identifying who carried out an attack is not as easy as it seems. When a regular soldier in full uniform with clear identification enters an MSF clinic and loots the place, MSF will usually say so unless this violates the "do no harm" principle. But these types of clear-cut situations are the exception rather than the rule. In many contexts, MSF is dealing with a multitude of armed groups, creating an environment where any security incident can easily be blamed on the "others," and often is.

This is also the case with aerial attacks. In Sudan, only one party has an air force—the Sudanese government—so there is no confusion about who did the bombing. This is similar for Gaza, where only the Israeli Defence Forces have this capacity. In Afghanistan it gets more muddled. Only the US-led alliance has airstrike capacity, so it is clear the armed opposition is not involved, but you cannot be precise in naming which air force is responsible, as multiple countries, including the Afghan government, are part of this military alliance, allowing a narrative of a "rogue action" within a complex hierarchy. MSF could be strong in its messaging about the perpetrator in the attack in Kunduz only because the United States immediately admitted that one of its planes was involved. Yemen is similar, with the Saudi-led coalition as the only air force at play. Unlike in Afghanistan, however, not a single nation of the Saudi-led coalition has taken responsibility for the airstrikes. This was reflected in MSF's statements, where blame was allocated to the "Saudi-led coalition" rather than to "Saudi Arabia." Iraq, with both an Iraqi air force and US-led coalition, is more ambiguous; MSF did not name perpetrators in this context, nor in Ukraine, where both Ukrainian and Russian air capacity was involved, using very similar planes and weaponry.

Syria is by far the messiest of these contexts, with two competing air coalitions and two nations unilaterally active in the skies over the country, all claiming to be bombing "terrorist" targets: the Syrian-led coalition, with a Syrian and Russian air force using very similar equipment; the US-led coalition, comprising the United States, France, the United Kingdom, Jordan, Bahrain, Qatar, Saudi Arabia, and other nations; Turkey, occasionally bombing Kurdish positions in Northern Syria; and Israel, bombing Iranian and Hezbollah targets around the country. Only the geographical location may indicate who is responsible for the attacks. The US coalition bombs only in Islamic State–controlled areas, so any location clearly outside this zone—such as Homs, Hama, or Damascus—is unlikely to involve the US-led coalition, although the Israeli air force is occasionally active there. In interface regions such as the Idlib and Aleppo governorates, where both competing air alliances are active, the situation is less clear-cut. And even if the alliance responsible can be identified, it is unlikely an untrained observer can spot which participating nation dropped bombs. Distinguishing between Syrian and Russian planes of the same make and model is almost impossible.

SHAMING

The shaming aspect is equally context sensitive. For Kunduz this was relatively straightforward, because the perpetrator was known by admission, and the destruction of a clearly marked hospital whose location was shared with all parties was witnessed by MSF employees (including international staff). A situation with little room for confusion, with credible witnesses and an environment where the protection of the hospital was explicitly agreed upon with the United States and all other warring parties. The same circumstances applied to Gaza in July 2015, although MSF stopped short of calling that attack a "presumed war crime" and stuck to "breach of IHL." For Kordofan, Sudan, MSF could have accused Sudan of breaching IHL. Although the Sudanese government did not explicitly agree with the establishment of the hospital, the building was marked, and its location was shared with the authorities in Khartoum. For some incidents MSF explicitly mentioned the sharing of GPS coordinates in its press statements, and in the case of the first hospital bombing in Yemen it even published a picture of the markings placed on the roof of the clinic. The Kunduz GPS coordinates became an iconic symbol marking some of MSF's publications about the event, to hammer home the message that IHL was breached.[17]

The paragraphs in IHL about the marking and notification of medical facilities are phrased as recommendations and options rather than obligations:

> The Parties to the conflict shall, in so far as military considerations permit, take the necessary steps to make the distinctive emblems indicating civilian hospitals clearly visible to the enemy land, air and naval forces in order to obviate the possibility of any hostile action. In view of the dangers to which hospitals may be exposed by being close to military objectives, it is recommended that such hospitals be situated as far as possible from such objectives. —Geneva Convention IV (1949), Article 18.[18]

International humanitarian law also specifies that the absence of these measures does not disqualify the hospital from protected status:

> The parties to the conflict are invited to notify each other of the location of their medical units. The absence of such notification shall not exempt any of the Parties from the obligation to comply with the provisions of paragraph 1 — Additional Protocol I (1977), Article 12.[19]

International humanitarian law does specify, however, how medical structures can lose their protected status:

> The protection to which fixed establishments and mobile medical units of the Medical Service are entitled shall not cease unless they are used to commit, outside their humanitarian duties, acts harmful to the enemy. Protection may, however, cease only after a due warning has been given, naming, in all appropriate cases, a reasonable time limit and after such warning has remained unheeded. —Geneva Convention I (1949), Article 21.[20]

So, although it is difficult to determine from IHL what precise measures the hospital must fulfill to gain protected status, it is clear from IHL that warring parties must notify a hospital when the belligerent believes protected status has been lost, and before military action is undertaken. In none of the 29 cases examined was MSF notified of the pending attacks, so technically, all the instances were a breach of IHL—indicating that the decision to accuse on grounds of IHL was not linked to the practice of marking and notification. The reason to mark and notify is more a common-sense self-interest. Even if only advised by IHL and not necessarily a legal obligation, common sense dictates that in demanding not to be targeted, you need to specify where you are. "I am hiding, but don't hit me anyway" does not work.

This explains why the case of Syria is the most ambiguous, showing an inconsistency in MSF's public positioning around hospital bombings that cannot be justified by context alone. By MSF's own admission, most of the health facilities were "underground" and "clandestine." From early in the conflict, persecution of medical staff for "illegally" treating wounded protesters set a trend for establishing "field hospitals," a euphemism for medical facilities that "were established in hidden places like basements, farm houses, deserted buildings, mosques, churches and factories" (Sankari et al. 2013).

HIDDEN HOSPITALS, POLITICAL MANIPULATION, AND REMOTE WITNESSING IN SYRIA

These specifics of the Syrian conflict put MSF—and other humanitarian witnesses—in an enormously vulnerable position. Syria is a high-profile conflict, with direct or indirect involvement of almost all regional and global powers. This puts any public positioning and witnessing in the spotlight and under scrutiny, especially from a big humanitarian brand like MSF. It also creates an environment in which it is nearly certain that any MSF public statement could be used by warring parties to support their own military narratives. Yet the reliability of MSF communications is easy to discredit: Are the partners MSF works with doctors first, or opposition activists first? Can the medical data provided by such partners be unbiased? Is MSF stating medical facts, or military propaganda?

These accusations are difficult to counter when MSF staff is not present on site and medical partners work in "underground" hospitals. Within MSF, the debate about this dilemma of "secondhand witnessing" often has taken an emotional turn around the argument that if MSF trusts these doctors to receive our medicines, we should trust the information they give us. The question, however, is not whether MSF trusts its medics—it is whether the warring parties trust these medics enough to allow them to bring in supplies and bring out the wounded. When information is easily manipulated, the warring parties' trust in MSF's medical colleagues is diminished. MSF never controls the output of what happens with a message, but in these cases of remote information-gathering, it also does not control the input of what goes into creating the message. Two cases of such manipulation illustrate this problem.

Case of Madaya

On January 7, 2016, MSF was the first medical agency to communicate about cases of starvation in a besieged area: "23 patients in the health centre supported by Médecins Sans Frontières (MSF) have died of starvation since 01 December."[21] Such a bold statement was always likely to be challenged by those imposing the siege. The cross-checking mechanisms MSF used relied exclusively on networks and partners operating on the antigovernment end of the political spectrum, organizations that also supplied medicines to the area: SAMS, The Union of Medical Care and Relief Organisations (UOMMS), and Qatar Red Crescent. MSF recognized this weakness in the cross-checking mechanism, and MSF made efforts to include Damascus-based medical organizations such as the Syrian Arab Red Crescent, the United Nations Children's Fund, ICRC, and WHO in the networks used for this purpose. This was only partially successful, because Damascus-based organizations were reluctant to share details. But it was sufficient to reveal the existence of this bias.

Madaya was a primary example where expanding the cross-checking networks exposed the risk of political bias, even with seemingly simple medical facts. Three weeks after the first press release, MSF communicated on January 29 that "The situation in Madaya is even worse as there are no doctors present in the town."[22] Conversations with ICRC and WHO, which both managed to visit Madaya (with international staff) after the alarming statements from MSF, found there were two doctors in a second, Ministry of Health–run, clinic in Madaya. When this information was checked with MSF's remote partners in Madaya, they replied, "Yes, we know, but we don't count them because the people don't trust them." For them, the question, "How many doctors?" meant "How many trusted doctors?"—and MSF lost some credibility as a result.

The attack of February 15, 2016, in Marat Al Numan, Idlib province, reignited the internal discussion in MSF on naming and shaming. Although MSF's official press release was rather bland and did not name a responsible party, Mego Terzian, President of MSF in Paris, did directly accuse the Syrian and Russian governments: "The author of the strike is clearly . . . either the government or Russia," adding that it was not the first time MSF facilities had been targeted in the country.[23] This was the first time MSF had directly accused Russia, and Russia forcefully denied the claim the next day, demanding "proof" and accusing the United States of responsibility.[24] Russia was able to make this claim because at that time, Marat Al Numan was controlled by the Al Nusra Brigade, an opposition group designated by Russia and the United States as an Al Qaeda affiliate and "terrorist" group, on both their lists of military targets.

Although MSF has strong legitimacy to provide medical assessments and data, it is not considered an expert on military hardware. To expect medical staff to identify an airplane high in the sky while running for their lives is not realistic. To overcome this problem, the WHO surveillance system recognized that "our system, however, does not feature specific expertise on weapons identification" by relying "on the experience of MVH partners, who, like much of the Syrian population, have grown familiar with different types of weaponry used by combatants," adding however that "similarly, the system does not conduct forensic investigation of the verified attacks" (Elamein 2017).

MSF nevertheless decided to go down this forensic path to counter Russia's denials of responsibility, engaging a UK-based organization, Forensic Architecture, to conduct an investigation into the bombings.[25] Forensic Architecture used pictures and video footage provided by residents around the town, as well as testimonies, to determine the exact timing, providence, and nature of the bombs and warplanes used. It concluded with near certainty that the MSF-supported hospital had been bombed by Russia, but that the other hospital in the town, bombed later that day, had been hit by the Syrian air force. Yet Forensic Architecture operates under similar constraints as MSF: It has no direct access to Syria, relying on third parties to provide footage and testimonies. Because the actual footage provided showed only a blur high in the sky, the most important evidence presented about the plane hitting the MSF-supported hospital was testimony by the "FSA observatory."[26] The FSA—Free Syrian Army—observes all Russian and Syrian airfields in Syria, marking the exact times planes take off. But as the FSA is an opposition force, Russia could easily dismiss its testimony as biased: the rebels were likely to accuse their enemies, not their allies.

THE LIMITED EFFECTS OF NAMING AND SHAMING

In the three years examined, MSF was fairly consistent in its discourse on perpetrators. For countries where there was no ambiguity—Sudan and Gaza, with only one air force active, plus Afghanistan and Yemen, by self-admission—MSF did not shy away from pointing the finger. In this logic the odd one out was Iraq, where MSF could have named the "Iraq-led coalition." Ukraine was too ambiguous to make that call. Syria was a muddle: confusion in the air with multiple and competing coalitions, combined with a perceived bias on the part of non-MSF medical partners on the ground as principle witnesses, working in largely unmarked and unnotified "field hospitals."

On the "shaming" side, MSF's record between 2014 and 2016 was more of a mixed bag. In nineteen of twenty-nine cases, MSF limited its accusations to a standard condemnation of "hitting patients and staff" and "depriving the population of essential healthcare," invoking a "breach of IHL" that was seemingly random. Part of the problem is that IHL as a concept is not universally supported within MSF. Opponents point out that IHL is limited in what is *not* allowed with regard to civilians and medical structures, but quite liberal in what *is* allowed: shoot, bomb, and destroy as you see fit, as long as you appear to "make an effort" to spare civilians and their structures, especially hospitals. In that sense IHL can and has been described as legitimizing the brutality of war rather than curtailing it (Madar 2012).

Supporters insist that IHL is the only international legal framework independent organizations such as MSF can call on to justify their own presence in war zones and make demands for access and protection, even though this legitimacy relies on the two words *"such as"* in Geneva Convention I (1949), Article 3: "An impartial humanitarian body, such as the International Committee of the Red Cross, may offer its services to the Parties to the conflict"[27]

In this logic, defending the continued application of IHL, however imperfect, is also a matter of self-interest and self-preservation for an organization such as MSF. With this duality about IHL in mind, it makes sense that MSF cried "IHL" after the Afghanistan, Yemen, and Gaza bombings—in the expectation that the parties concerned might be convinced by invoking their obligations under IHL—but did not do so in the cases of Iraq, Sudan, and Ukraine, where the expectations about the respect for IHL were more limited.

Syria, in this logic, should be the country with the lowest expectation of any respect for IHL—it is a place where disregard for the sanctity of the medical act during war is so low that medics feel forced to go underground in makeshift, unmarked hospitals in secret locations. This in turn allows the bombers to claim these hospitals are not protected, because their hidden nature "proves" they are used for military purposes. Yet MSF still claimed "breach of IHL" in five of seventeen events between 2014 and 2016. This claim, however, was not made on the same basis as in Afghanistan, Gaza, and Yemen: that a warring party, in breach of IHL, targeted a clearly marked hospital. In Syria it was a condemnation of the overall brutality of the war.

In East Aleppo, Idlib, East Ghouta, and Homs, everything was bombed: schools, mosques, markets, houses, and hospitals. MSF-managed or MSF-supported hospitals dealt with the consequences, treating hundreds or thousands of wounded in each case. MSF published a report with a documented analysis of the medical and humanitarian consequences of the intensification of the military campaign in 2015, based on medical reports and data from seventy clinics and hospitals in Syria supported by MSF:

> The findings are particularly concerning because the 70 makeshift hospitals and clinics that are regularly supported by MSF constitute only a small fraction of the health facilities in Syria. The large number of dead (7,009 people) and wounded (154,647 people) recorded in this report represents the people who were able to reach a health facility and does not account for deaths outside the clinics or wounded who were unable to reach a facility. . . . Particularly concerning is that, in 2015, women and children represented between 30 and 40 percent of the victims of violence in Syria, indicating that civilian areas were consistently hit by aerial bombardments and other forms of attack. (MSF 2016)

In four of the ninety-eight attacks recorded in 2015, the report found use of a "double tap" strategy—returning to the scene of an attack for a second bombardment after the medical workers have arrived—which may indicate intent to single out health care. But it generally concluded that, whether intentional on health care or indiscriminate against civilians, IHL had been breached. MFS's language also became more precise: before Syria, the terms "hit" and "targeted" were used interchangeably; but with Syria "targeted" was phased out, because it implied specific intent on a hospital, which sounded hollow when a whole neighbourhood was flattened. For Syria, the indiscriminate nature of the attacks—the clear lack of any attempt to avoid hitting civilians and civilian infrastructure—prompted MSF to claim breaches of IHL in most cases.

The report was addressed directly to the UN Security Council, noting that in 2015, four out of the five permanent members (the United States, Russia, the United Kingdom, and France) were actively participating in this war—something that had happened only once before, during the Korean War of the 1950s (where it was China, not Russia, joining the other three). This observation was later used by the president of MSF in her speech to the UN Security Council in February 2016: "Four of the five permanent members of the UN Security Council are involved in military operations in Syria. They are failing to abide by their own resolutions protecting civilians, healthcare, and the provision of humanitarian assistance."[28] The Security Council subsequently adopted Resolution 2286 and issued a statement "strongly condemning attacks on medical personnel in conflict situations today." The council went on to demand "an end to impunity for those responsible and respect for international law on the part of all warring parties."[29] The four permanent members were seemingly oblivious to the irony that they were effectively condemning themselves. Unsurprisingly, the practice of hospital bombings did not diminish in Syria—its most brutal episode, in East Aleppo, still to come at the end of 2016.

The debate at the UN Security Council in February 2016, where both ICRC and MSF were invited to speak, represented the peak of international attention and pressure, especially on states, to stop the practice of hospital bombings. Looking at Syria alone, this had no impact—attacks continued undiminished, reduced only as a function of the amount of territory controlled by armed opposition groups. By 2019, rebels controlled only one small region around Idlib, so in absolute numbers the number of attacks went down, though in proportion to the size of the region, not by much. Globally the number of aerial attacks on hospitals—in all cases, attacks by states—has decreased as well, and not only as a result of changing conflict dynamics. The conflicts in Yemen and Afghanistan continue without much respite, yet hospitals have not been bombed there for some time. This may give hope that naming and shaming have had an effect, at least in some countries.

History shows that states rarely hold themselves to account, preferring to deflect blame and question the legitimacy of the medical action. Public pressure can make a difference, and humanitarians can play a crucial role in generating such pressure. But faith in humanitarian organizations requires that they offer strong, consistent, and accurate accounts of events, something MSF and others drifted away from in Syria, as access was restricted by the Syrian government and by security threats from the opposition. This allowed the bombing states, Syria and Russia, to discredit MSF's accounts to their allies at home and abroad with relative ease— and never feel any pressure to stop their aerial assaults. In Syria, naming and shaming to stop hospital bombings has failed.

NOTES

1. http://www.emro.who.int/media/news/who-condemns-attack-on-abs-hospital-and-calls-for-protection-of-health-staff-and-facilities-in-yemen.html
2. https://www.msf.org/kunduz-hospital-attack-depth
3. https://healthcareindanger.org/
4. https://www.msf.org/medical-care-under-fire
5. WHO Surveillance System for Attacks on Healthcare (SSA): https://extranet.who.int/ssa/Index.aspx
6. https://ihl-databases.icrc.org/ihl/INTRO/120
7. See Chapter 7 of this volume by Alexey Khlebnikov
8. https://undocs.org/S/RES/2286(2016)
9. https://www.msf.org/syria-eastern-aleppo-hospitals-damaged-23-attacks-july
10. https://www.aljazeera.com/news/2016/09/syria-ceasefire-effect-russia-deal-160912125315496.html
11. https://www.doctorswithoutborders.org/what-we-do/news-stories/news/msf-condemns-bombing-its-hospital-kajo-keji-southern-sudan
12. http://www.msf.org/article/msf-hospital-bombed-sudan
13. http://www.msf.org/article/afghanistan-msf-staff-killed-and-hospital-partially-destroyed-kunduz
14. 19 Nov. 2016: https://www.msf.org/syria-multiple-direct-and-indirect-hits-hospitals-east-aleppo-last-48-hours
    17 Nov. 2016: https://www.msf.org/syria-hospital-bombings-east-aleppo-force-staff-move-children-and-premature-babies-basement-shelter
    15 Oct. 2016: https://www.msf.org/syria-latest-attacks-east-aleppo-hospitals-leave-medical-care-tatters
    7 Oct. 2016: https://www.msf.org/syria-four-hospitals-hit-bombing-and-shelling-continue-damascus-region
    7 Oct. 2016: https://www.msf.org/syria-eastern-aleppo-hospitals-damaged-23-attacks-july
    5 Oct. 2016: https://www.msf.org/syria-hospitals-hit-repeatedly-russian-and-syrian-airstrikes-condemning-hundreds-wounded-certain
    30 Sept. 2016: https://www.msf.org/syria-msf-urges-syrian-government-and-its-allies-stop-indiscriminate-bombing-aleppo
    28 Sept. 2016: https://www.msf.org/syria-two-surgical-hospitals-bombed-east-aleppo
    15 Aug. 2016: https://www.msf.org/yemen-eleven-people-dead-and-least-19-injured-after-airstrike-hits-abs-hospital-hajjah
    8 Aug. 2016: https://www.msf.org/syria-msf-supported-hospital-idlib-bombed-ground-amid-increased-intensity-attacks
    28 April 2016: https://www.msf.org/syria-airstrike-destroys-msf-supported-hospital-aleppo-killing-14
    15 Feb. 2016: https://www.msf.org/syria-least-11-killed-another-msf-supported-hospital-attack-idlib-province

9 Feb. 2016: https://www.msf.org/syria-msf-supported-hospital-hit-airstrikes

10 Jan. 2016: https://www.msf.org/
   msf-supported-hospital-bombed-yemen-death-toll-rises-six

3 Dec. 2015: http://www.msf.org/article/
   yemen-nine-wounded-saudi-led-coalition-airstrike-msf-clinic-taiz

1 Dec. 2015: http://www.msf.org/article/syria-double-tap-bombing-
   msf-supported-hospital-%E2%80%93-hospital-partially-destroyed-
   %E2%80%93-patients

21 Nov. 2015: http://www.msf.org/article/
   syria-msf-appalled-another-supported-hospital-damascus-area-hit-missiles

27 Oct. 2015: http://www.msf.org/article/
   yemen-msf-hospital-destroyed-airstrikes

3 Oct. 2015: http://www.msf.org/article/
   afghanistan-msf-staff-killed-and-hospital-partially-destroyed-kunduz

14 Aug. 2015: http://www.msf.org/article/syria-airstrikes-nine-hospitals-idlib-
   province-11-civilians-killed-and-31-wounded

18 June 2015: http://www.msf.org/article/
   syria-barrage-barrel-bombs-destroys-msf-health-facility

4 May 2015: http://www.msf.org/article/
   syria-main-hospital-aleppo-stops-activities-after-being-targeted

3 Feb. 2015: http://www.doctorswithoutborders.org/article/
   ukraine-msf-expanding-aid-efforts-shelling-hospitals-continues

23 Jan. 2015: http://www.doctorswithoutborders.org/article/
   ukraine-hospitals-shelled-and-civilians-cut-fighting-intensifies

22 Jan. 2015: http://www.msf.org/article/
   sudan-msf-hospital-bombed-south-kordofan

29 July 2014: http://www.msf.org/article/
   msf-strongly-condemns-attack-al-shifa-hospital

24 July 2014: http://www.msf.org/article/
   iraq-hospitals-destroyed-air-strikes-leave-iraqis-without-healthcare

18 June 2014: http://www.msf.org/article/
   iraq-msf-calls-respect-medical-facilities

17 June 2014: http://www.msf.org/article/msf-hospital-bombed-sudan

15. https://apnews.com/article/c545c1533d1344878f6bd027e9e9f9a0; https://
   www.bbc.co.uk/news/world-middle-east-35586886

16. "The IHFFC is the dedicated expert body established by Additional Protocol I to
   the Geneva Conventions to respond to incidents in relation to international
   humanitarian law. It stands at the service of parties to an armed conflict to
   conduct enquiries into alleged violations and to facilitate, through its good
   offices, the restoration of an attitude of respect for that body of law." —
   Introduction on IHFFC home page. www.ihffc.org.

17. https://www.msf.org/kunduz-afghanistan-36°43'491"n-68°51'4396"

18. ICRC, Customary IHL Database: https://www.icrc.org/customary-ihl/eng/docs/
   v2_rul_rule28

19. ICRC, Customary IHL Database: https://www.icrc.org/customary-ihl/eng/docs/
   v2_rul_rule28

20. ICRC, Customary IHL Database: https://www.icrc.org/customary-ihl/eng/docs/
   v2_rul_rule28

21. https://www.msf.org/syria-siege-and-starvation-madaya-immediate-medical-
   evacuations-and-medical-resupply-essential-save

22. https://www.msf.org/syria-starvation-continues-madaya-msf-denounces-continued-blockage-essential-aid-and-medical
23. https://uk.reuters.com/article/us-mideast-crisis-syria-missiles/around-50-dead-as-missiles-hit-medical-centers-and-schools-in-syrian-towns-idUKKCN0VO12Y
24. https://www.bbc.co.uk/news/world-middle-east-35586886
25. https://forensic-architecture.org/investigation/airstrikes-on-al-hamidiah-hospital
26. Ibid.
27. ICRC, Customary IHL Database: https://ihl-databases.icrc.org/ihl/WebART/365-570006
28. https://www.msf.org/syria-statement-dr-joanne-liu-international-president-médecins-sans-frontières
29. https://www.un.org/press/en/2016/sc12347.doc.htm

REFERENCES

Abu Sa'Da, Caroline, Françoise Duroch, and Bertrand Taithe. 2013. "Attacks on Medical Missions: Overview of a Polymorphous Reality: The case of Médecins Sans Frontières." *International Review of the Red Cross* 95 (890): 309–30. doi:10.1017/S1816383114000186.

Atlantic Council. 2017. "Breaking Aleppo." Atlantic Council. https://www.publications.atlanticcouncil.org/breakingaleppo/.

Barnett, Michael. 2011. *Empire of Humanity: A History of Humanitarianism*. Ithaca, NY: Cornell University Press.

Bouchet-Saulnier, Françoise, and Jonathan Whittall. 2018. "An Environment Conducive to Mistakes? Lessons Learnt From the Attack on the Médecins Sans Frontières Hospital in Kunduz, Afghanistan." *International Review of the Red Cross* 100 (907–09): 337–72. doi:10.1017/S1816383118000619.

Briody, Carolyn, Leonard Rubenstein, Les Roberts, Eamon Penney, William Keenan, and Jeffrey Horbar. 2018. "Review of Attacks on Health Care Facilities in Six Conflicts of the Past Three Decades." *Conflict and Health* 12 (19). doi:10.1186/s13031-018-0152-2.

Elamein, Mohamed, Hilary Bower, Camilo Valderrama, Daher Zedan, Hazem Rihawi, Khaled Almilaji, Mohammed Abdelhafeez, Nabil Tabbal, Naser Almhawish, Sophie Maes and Alaa AbouZeid. 2017. "Attacks Against Health Care in Syria, 2015–16: Results From a Real-Time Reporting Tool." *Lancet* 390 (10109): 2278–86. doi:10.1016/S0140-6736(17)31328-4.

Fouad, Fouad M., Annie Sparrow, Ahmad Tarakji, Mohamad Alameddine, Fadi El-Jardali, Adam P Coutts, Nour El Arnaout, Lama Bou Karroum, Mohammed Jawad, Sophie Roborgh, Aula Abbara, Fadi Alhalabi, Ibrahim AlMasri and, Samer Jabbour. 2017. "Health Workers and the Weaponisation of Health Care in Syria: A Preliminary Inquiry for *The Lancet*–American University of Beirut Commission on Syria." *Lancet* 390 (10111): 2516–26. doi:10.1016/S0140-6736(17)30741-9.

Madar, Chase. 2012. "Do 'Laws of War' Simply Legitimize 'War Crimes'?" *Common Dreams*. https://www.commondreams.org/views/2012/04/16/do-laws-war-simply-legitimize-war-crimes.

McLean, Duncan. 2019. "Medical Care in Armed Conflict: Perpetrator Discourse in Historical Perspective." *International Review of the Red Cross* 101 (911): 771–803. doi:10.1017/S1816383120000016.

MSF (Médecins Sans Frontières). 2012. "Syria: Medicine as a Weapon of Persecution." MSF. https://www.msf.org/syria-medicine-used-weapon-persecution.

MSF (Médecins Sans Frontières). 2016. "Syria 2015: Documenting War-Wounded and War -Dead in MSF-Supported Medical Facilities in Syria." MSF. https://www.msf.org/sites/msf.org/files/2018-05/syria_2015_war-dead_and_war-wounded_report_en.pdf.

OHCHR (Office of the United Nations High Commissioner for Human Rights). 2013. "Assault on Medical Care in Syria." OHCHR. https://www.ohchr.org/EN/HRBodies/HRC/RegularSessions/Session24/Documents/A-HRC-24-CRP-2.doc.

PHR (Physicians for Human Rights). 2019. "The Syrian Conflict: Eight Years of Devastation and Destruction of the Health System." PHR. https://phr.org/our-work/resources/the-syrian-conflict-eight-years-of-devastation-and-destruction-of-the-health-system/.

Safeguarding Health in Conflict. 2017. "Impunity Must End: Attacks on Health in 23 Countries in Conflict in 2016." Safeguarding Health in Conflict. https://www.safeguardinghealth.org/sites/shcc/files/SHCC2017final.pdf.

SAMS (Syrian American Medical Society). 2017. "The Failure of UN Security Council Resolution 2286 in Preventing Attacks on Healthcare in Syria." SAMS. https://www.sams-usa.net/reports/failure-un-security-council-resolution-2286-preventing-attacks-healthcare-syria/.

Sankari, Abdulghani, Basel Atassi, and Mohammed Zaher Sahloul. 2013. "Syrian Field Hospitals: A Creative Solution in Urban Military Conflict Combat in Syria." *Avicenna Journal of Medicine* 3 (3): 84–86. doi:10.4103/2231-0770.118467.

UNGA (United Nations General Assembly) Human Rights Council. 2017. "Report of the Independent International Commission of Inquiry on the Syrian Arab Republic." UNGA. https://undocs.org/A/HRC/34/64.

WHO (World Health Organization). 2016. "Report on Attacks on Health Care in Emergencies." WHO. https://www.who.int/hac/techguidance/attacksreport.pdf.

INDEX

Note: Tables and figures are indicated by *t* and *f* following the page number

Hezbollah, 140–141, 192, 193, 199
Higher Defence Council, 144
Hobbes, Thomas, 79
hospital attacks/bombings
  acceleration of, 190–191
  in Afghanistan, 185, 194, 195, 198, 205
  after 2010, 188–190
  Geneva Conventions historical
    limitations, 186–188
  introduction to, 8, 34, 77, 185–186
  Médecins sans Frontières and, 173–174,
    185–186, 194–199
  military hospitals, 42, 65, 73
  naming and shaming perpetrators,
    192–194, 198–207
  public hospitals, 15, 42, 45, 62, 64, 96
  by Russia, 75–76, 176, 185, 190,
    192–195
  by Saudi Arabia, 185, 190, 194, 199
  by Syrian government, 27, 67, 174,
    178, 190–193
  by United States, 185
  university hospitals, 42
  in Yemen, 185, 188–189, 194, 197–
    198, 200–206, 205
House of Commons Foreign Affairs
  Select Committee (UK), 170
Howell, Alison, 70
human dignity concerns, 68, 148
human rights
  abuses and violations, 59, 60, 77,
    168–170
  domestic criminal law and, 65
  humanitarianism after cold war, 187
  international human rights law, 27, 58
  legal advocacy and, 78–81
  manufacturing vulnerability, 145
  military involvement and, 161
  sanctions and, 149
  siege warfare and, 138
human rights organizations, 59, 60,
  68, 77, 188–189. *See also* specific
  organizations
Human Rights Watch (HRW), 80, 144, 171
humanitarian aid. *See also* siege
    experiences of refugees
  accumulation of wealth and, 115–116
  aid-related dilemmas, 125–127
  aid to opposition-controlled areas,
    120–121

besiegement and, 2, 122–125
broader aid system in question,
  127–128
consensus on meaning of, 131n1
cross-border delivery of, 47–48
economics of state survival, 113–114
future challenges, 130–131
government-sanctioned aid, 117–120
importance of, 128–130
introduction to, 2, 8, 111–112
lack of transparency, 39, 41
limits of, 5–6
pre-uprising antecedents, 112–113
restrictions to, 1–2, 4–5
self-defeating sanctions, 116–117
shared failures, 10–12
humanitarian complicity in sieges,
  152–155
hypertension rates, 35

IHH (Humanitarian Relief Foundation),
  103, 106
Independent International Commission
  of Inquiry, 62
India, 162, 165
infant mortality, 18
information warfare, 168, 170–173
institutional humanitarianism, 160–161
Inter-Agency Standing Committee,
  180n4
Inter-War French mandate over Syria, 87
Intermediate-Range Nuclear Forces
  (INF) treaty, 162
internally displaced people (IDPs), 44–
  45, 47, 167
International Civil Defense Organization
  (ICDO), 171
International Committee of the Red
  Cross (ICRC), 4, 43, 68, 74, 76, 152,
  171, 187, 202, 204
International Crisis Group (ICG), 102
International Federation of Red Cross, 43
international financial organizations
  (IFOs), 21
international human rights law, 27, 58, 144
International Humanitarian Fact Finding
  Commission (IHFFC), 197
international humanitarian law (IHL)
  breach of, 187, 197–198, 200–201,
  204–205

United States (US)
  aid contributions by, 129
  assistance to Jordan, 100
  bombing by, 140–142, 194–195, 198–199
  exports to Syria, 148
  field manual on siege warfare, 136–138
  hospital bombings by, 185
  invasion of Iraq, 3, 80
  military doctrine, 139
  in political coalitions, 93, 154, 173, 177–178, 193, 199
  sanctions by, 148–149
  troop withdrawals, 45
  war on terror, 27, 139
university hospitals, 42

vaccination campaigns, 15
Van Schaack, Beth, 138
Vietnam War, 80
Vietnamese "boat people," 108
Violations Documentation Center in Syria, 36

war crimes, 45, 58, 68, 117, 170, 191
war on terror, 27, 139
"Wasta" (connections), 43
water, sanitation, and hygiene (WASH) damages, 46, 49, 50
"weaponization" of health care, 191
welfare-provision sectors, 21
Western humanitarian actors, 14
White Helmets, 171–172
World Bank, 98
World Food Programme (WFP), 151–152
World Health Organization (WHO), 19, 37, 43, 78, 171, 185, 189, 202
World Trade Organization, 162
World War I, 87

Yarubieh border crossing closure, 44
Yemen, hospital bombings in, 185, 188–189, 194, 197–198, 200–206, 205

Za'tari refugee camp, 89–90, 97–98
Zerofsky, Elisabeth, 147